MW00593791

90-DAY FITNESS JOURNAL

YOUR COMPLETE FITNESS COMPANION

ROSE SERY

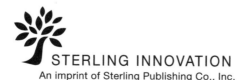

STERLING INNOVATION
An imprint of Sterling Publishing Co., Inc.

New York / London
www.sterlingpublishing.com

STERLING, the Sterling logo, STERLING INNOVATION, and the Sterling
Innovation logo are registered trademarks of Sterling Publishing Co., Inc.

10 9 8 7 6 5 4 3 2

Published by Sterling Publishing Co., Inc.
387 Park Avenue South, New York, NY 10016
© 2009 by Sterling Publishing Co., Inc.

Distributed in Canada by Sterling Publishing
c/o Canadian Manda Group, 165 Dufferin Street
Toronto, Ontario, Canada M6K 3H6
Distributed in the United Kingdom by GMC Distribution Services
Castle Place, 166 High Street, Lewes, East Sussex, England BN7 1XU
Distributed in Australia by Capricorn Link (Australia) Pty. Ltd.
P.O. Box 704, Windsor, NSW 2756, Australia

Sterling ISBN 978-1-4027-6755-5

For information about custom editions, special sales, premium and
corporate purchases, please contact Sterling Special Sales Department
at 800-805-5489 or specialsales@sterlingpublishing.com.

Nothing tastes as good as being healthy feels.
—Anonymous

CONTENTS

GETTING HEALTHY

Did you know that about two-thirds of American adults are overweight? All those extra pounds not only make us feel self-conscious, but they can lead to serious health problems such as diabetes, high blood pressure, and even certain kinds of cancer. It's time to take your weight and measurements into your own hands and get healthy.

This journal is your all-inclusive guide to healthier living. It will help you set realistic and healthy goals for weight loss, track your diet and exercise progress over the next 90 days, and keep you on the road to fitness and a healthier life for years to come.

GOALS

The first step to weight loss is setting goals. On page 11 you will find a Body Mass Index, or BMI, chart that will show you a healthy weight for your height. Your goal weight should fall in the normal range. However, healthy weight loss averages 2 pounds per week, so don't set your goals too high, or too low. It may take you more than 90 days to reach your ideal weight, it may take less. Your real goal is to discover a healthy lifestyle that will help you reach your desired weight and keep you there.

EATING

The next step is to understand your current eating behavior—and then to change it. To maintain your current weight you have to consume about 12 to 15 calories per day for every pound you weigh. So if you weigh 175 pounds, you need to eat 2,100 to 2,625 calories per day to stay there. If you want to lose weight, then you have to eat fewer calories. If you want to lose about 1 pound per week, you should reduce your calorie intake by about 500 calories per day. If you want to lose twice that, then you need to reduce your calorie intake by 1,000 calories per day. But don't push it too far! Women should eat at least 1,200 calories per day, and men should eat 1,500 to maintain a healthy diet.

Fats, carbohydrates, and protein are three of the most important energy producing nutrients for the human body, but that doesn't mean you should overdo it. Reducing the amount of fats and carbohydrates you eat is a great way to cut down on calorie consumption and promote healthy weight loss, because they are not only high in calories but low in vitamins and minerals too.

To launch an overall healthier lifestyle, you should make sure you are getting all of the recommended vitamins and minerals and not eating "empty calories"—foods that have no nutritional value and are high in fat, carbs, and calories. Eating as little saturated fat as possible will lead to weight loss and healthy gains. Getting your daily protein from lean meats, soy, cheese, yogurt, and eggs is a very healthy way to go, because each food has additional nutritional value above being high in protein.

To figure out your daily balance of calories and fats, use the formulas on pages 20–21.

At the back of this journal is an extensive list of common foods, their calorie contents, and their fat contents. This guide will help you keep track of your daily fat and caloric intake when eating out or when you don't have a nutritional label on your food. Also included are charts that show the recommended intakes of vitamins and minerals, as well as lists of healthy foods that contain daily essentials. By using this information, you can construct a diet to help you lose weight, stay in good health, and eat foods you love.

WATER

People often overlook the importance of water in planning a healthy diet. There are realms of reasons why drinking water is great for everyone. People who drink eight 8-ounce glasses of water every day lose weight faster than people who don't, because water speeds up metabolic processes, helping you shed stored fat. It also moves waste and fat out of your body. Like oil in an engine, water keeps your body moving.

EXERCISE

The final step to a healthier you is exercise. Daily exercise will help you lose weight; strengthen your muscles, heart, and lungs; and give you more energy. Finding the right exercise for you is extremely important. First, take any health issues into consideration. Then, you need to find an aerobic activity that you enjoy. Exercise doesn't have to be a chore or a bore. Find a scenic place to walk, join a gym and learn karate, or discover that you're a natural tennis player. If you find an exercise you love, you'll stick with it and really enjoy your road to healthier living.

On pages 13–19 you will find a chart showing how many calories you burn per hour doing a variety of exercises.

A NEW YOU!

Leading a healthful life is the best thing you can do for yourself, and looking and feeling better for the rest of your life is only 90 days away. Being conscious of the things you put into your body and do with your body is the only way to diet effectively and healthily. This journal will help you become aware of the things you're already doing that help or hurt you, and will guide you to better way of living. Get ready, because in 90 days there will be a whole new you!

BMI CHART[1]

BMI	19	20	21	22	23	24	25	26	27	28	29	30	31	32	33	34	35

HEIGHT   WEIGHT IN POUNDS

HEIGHT	19	20	21	22	23	24	25	26	27	28	29	30	31	32	33	34	35
4'10"	91	96	100	105	110	115	119	124	129	134	138	143	148	153	158	162	167
4'11"	94	99	104	109	114	119	124	128	133	138	143	148	153	158	163	168	173
5'	97	102	107	112	118	123	128	133	138	143	148	153	158	163	158	174	179
5'1"	100	106	111	116	122	127	132	137	143	148	153	158	164	169	174	180	185
5'2"	104	109	115	120	126	131	136	142	147	153	158	164	169	175	180	186	191
5'3"	107	113	118	124	130	135	141	146	152	158	163	169	175	180	186	191	197
5'4"	110	116	122	128	134	140	145	151	157	163	169	174	180	186	192	197	204
5'5"	114	120	126	132	138	144	150	156	162	168	174	180	186	192	198	204	210
5'6"	118	124	130	136	142	148	155	161	167	173	179	186	192	198	204	210	216
5'7"	121	127	134	140	146	153	159	166	172	178	185	191	198	204	211	217	223
5'8"	125	131	138	144	151	158	164	171	177	184	190	197	203	210	216	223	230
5'9"	128	135	142	149	155	162	169	176	182	189	196	203	209	216	223	230	236
5'10"	132	139	146	153	160	167	174	181	188	195	202	209	216	222	229	236	243
5'11"	136	143	150	157	165	172	179	186	193	200	208	215	222	229	236	243	250
6'	140	147	154	162	169	177	184	191	199	206	213	221	228	235	242	250	258
6'1"	144	151	159	166	174	182	189	197	204	212	219	227	235	242	250	257	265
6'2"	148	155	163	171	179	186	194	202	210	218	225	233	241	249	256	264	272
6'3"	152	160	168	176	184	192	200	208	216	224	232	240	248	256	264	272	279
	HEALTHY WEIGHT						OVERWEIGHT					OBESE					

1. Dietary Guidelines for Americans 2005
   U.S. Department of Health and Human Services
   U.S. Department of Agriculture
   www.healthierus.gov/dietaryguidelines

EXERCISE CHART

ESTIMATED CALORIES BURNED PER HOUR BASED ON BODY WEIGHT[2]

	130 LBS.	155 LBS.	190 LBS.
Aerobics, general	354	422	518
Aerobics, high impact	413	493	604
Aerobics, low impact	295	352	431
Archery (non-hunting)	207	246	302
Automobile repair	177	211	259
Backpacking, general	413	493	604
Badminton, competitive	413	493	604
Badminton, social, general	266	317	388
Basketball, game	472	563	690
Basketball, non-game, general	354	422	518
Basketball, officiating	413	493	604
Basketball, shooting baskets	266	317	388
Basketball, wheelchair	384	457	561
Bicycling, < 10 mph, leisure	236	281	345
Bicycling, > 20 mph, racing	944	1,126	1,380
Bicycling, 10-11.9 mph, light effort	354	422	518
Bicycling, 12-13.9 mph, moderate effort	472	563	690
Bicycling, 14-15.9 mph, vigorous effort	590	704	863
Bicycling, 16-19 mph, very fast, racing	708	844	1035
Bicycling, BMX or mountain	502	598	733
Bicycling, stationary, general	295	352	431
Bicycling, stationary, light effort	325	387	474
Bicycling, stationary, moderate effort	413	493	604
Bicycling, stationary, very light effort	177	211	259

2. Department of Health and Family Services
Division of Public Health
PPH 40109 (09/05)
dhs.wisconsin.gov/Health/physicalactivity/pdf_files/Caloriesperhour.pdf

	130 LBS.	155 LBS.	190 LBS.
Bicycling, stationary, very vigorous effort	738	880	1,078
Bicycling, stationary, vigorous effort	620	739	906
Billiards	148	176	216
Bowling	177	211	259
Boxing, in ring, general	708	844	1,035
Boxing, punching bag	354	422	518
Boxing, sparring	531	633	776
Broomball	413	493	604
Calisthenics (push-ups, sit-ups), vigorous effort	472	563	690
Calisthenics, home, light/moderate effort	266	317	388
Canoeing, on camping trip	236	281	345
Canoeing, rowing, > 6 mph, vigorous effort	708	844	1,035
Canoeing, rowing, crewing, competition	708	844	1,035
Canoeing, rowing, light effort	177	211	259
Canoeing, rowing, moderate effort	413	493	604
Carpentry, general	207	246	302
Carrying heavy loads, such as bricks	472	563	690
Child care: sitting, kneeling, dressing, feeding	177	211	259
Child care: standing-dressing, feeding	207	246	302
Circuit training, general	472	563	690
Cleaning, heavy, vigorous effort	266	317	388
Cleaning, house, general	207	246	302
Cleaning, light, moderate effort	148	176	216
Coaching: football, soccer, basketball, etc.	236	281	345
Construction, outside, remodeling	325	387	474
Cooking or food preparation	148	176	216
Cricket (batting, bowling)	295	352	431
Croquet	148	176	216
Curling	236	281	345

EXERCISE CHART

	130 LBS.	155 LBS.	190 LBS.
Dancing, aerobic, ballet or modern, twist	354	422	518
Dancing, ballroom, fast	325	387	474
Dancing, ballroom, slow	177	211	259
Dancing, general	266	317	388
Darts, wall or lawn	148	176	216
Diving, springboard or platform	177	211	259
Electrical work, plumbing	207	246	302
Farming, baling hay, cleaning barn	472	563	690
Farming, milking by hand	177	211	259
Farming, shoveling grain	325	387	474
Fencing	354	422	518
Fishing from boat, sitting	148	176	216
Fishing from river bank, standing	207	246	302
Fishing in stream, in waders	354	422	518
Fishing, general	236	281	345
Fishing, ice, sitting	118	141	173
Football or baseball, playing catch	148	176	216
Football, competitive	531	633	776
Football, touch, flag, general	472	563	690
Frisbee playing, general	177	211	259
Frisbee, ultimate	207	246	302
Gardening, general	295	352	431
Golf, carrying clubs	325	387	474
Golf, general	236	281	345
Golf, miniature or driving range	177	211	259
Golf, pulling clubs	295	352	431
Golf, using power cart	207	246	302
Gymnastics, general	236	281	345
Hacky sack	236	281	345

| --- | --- | --- | --- |
Handball, general	708	844	1,035
Handball, team	472	563	690
Hiking, cross country	354	422	518
Hockey, field	472	563	690
Hockey, ice	472	563	690
Horse grooming	354	422	518
Horse racing, galloping	472	563	690
Horseback riding, general	236	281	345
Horseback riding, trotting	384	457	561
Horseback riding, walking	148	176	216
Hunting, general	295	352	431
Jai alai	708	844	1,035
Jogging, general	413	493	604
Judo, karate, kick boxing, tae kwan do	590	704	863
Kayaking	295	352	431
Kickball	413	493	604
Lacrosse	472	563	690
Marching band, playing instrument (walking)	236	281	345
Marching, rapidly, military	384	457	561
Motocross	236	281	345
Moving furniture, household	354	422	518
Moving household items, boxes, upstairs	531	633	776
Moving household items, carrying boxes	413	493	604
Mowing lawn, general	325	387	474
Mowing lawn, riding mower	148	176	216
Music playing, cello, flute, horn, woodwind	118	141	173
Music playing, drums	236	281	345
Music playing, guitar, classical, folk (sitting)	118	141	173
Music playing, guitar, rock/roll band (standing)	177	211	259

EXERCISE CHART

	130 LBS.	155 LBS.	190 LBS.
Music playing, piano, organ, violin, trumpet	148	176	216
Paddleboat	236	281	345
Painting, papering, plastering, scraping	266	317	388
Polo	472	563	690
Pushing or pulling stroller with child	148	176	216
Race walking	384	457	561
Racquetball, casual, general	413	493	604
Racquetball, competitive	590	704	863
Raking lawn	236	281	345
Rock climbing, ascending rock	649	774	949
Rock climbing, rappelling	472	563	690
Rope jumping, fast	708	844	1,035
Rope jumping, moderate, general	590	704	863
Rope jumping, slow	472	563	690
Rowing, stationary, light effort	561	669	819
Rowing, stationary, moderate effort	413	493	604
Rowing, stationary, very vigorous effort	708	844	1035
Rowing, stationary, vigorous effort	502	598	733
Rugby	590	704	863
Running, 10 mph (6-min. mile)	944	1,126	1,380
Running, 10.9 mph (5.5-min. mile)	1,062	1,267	1,553
Running, 5 mph (12-min. mile)	472	563	690
Running, 5.2 mph (11.5-min. mile)	531	633	776
Running, 6 mph (10-min. mile)	590	704	863
Running, 6.7 mph (9-min. mile)	649	774	949
Running, 7 mph (8.5-min. mile)	679	809	992
Running, 7.5 mph (8-min. mile)	738	880	1,078
Running, 8 mph (7.5-min. mile)	797	950	1,165
Running, 8.6 mph (7-min. mile)	826	985	1,208

	130 LBS.	155 LBS.	190 LBS.
Running, 9 mph (6.5-min. mile)	885	1,056	1,294
Running, cross country	531	633	776
Running, general	472	563	690
Running, in place	472	563	690
Running, on a track, team practice	590	704	863
Running, stairs, up	885	1,056	1,294
Running, training, pushing wheelchair	472	563	690
Running, wheeling, general	177	211	259
Sailing, boat/board, windsurfing, general	177	211	259
Sailing, in competition	295	352	431
Scrubbing floors, on hands and knees	325	387	474
Shoveling snow, by hand	354	422	518
Shuffleboard, lawn bowling	177	211	259
Sitting-playing with children, light effort	148	176	216
Skateboarding	295	352	431
Skating, ice, 9 mph or less	325	387	474
Skating, ice, general	413	493	604
Skating, ice, rapidly, > 9 mph	531	633	776
Skating, ice, speed, competitive	885	1,056	1,294
Skating, roller	413	493	604
Ski jumping (climb up carrying skis)	413	493	604
Ski machine, general	561	669	819
Skiing, cross-country, > 8.0 mph, racing	826	985	1,208
Skiing, cross-country, moderate effort	472	563	690
Skiing, cross-country, slow or light effort	413	493	604
Skiing, cross-country, uphill, maximum effort	974	1,161	1,423
Skiing, cross-country, vigorous effort	531	633	776
Skiing, downhill, light effort	295	352	431
Skiing, downhill, moderate effort	354	422	518

EXERCISE CHART

	130 LBS.	155 LBS.	190 LBS.
Skiing, downhill, vigorous effort, racing	472	563	690
Skiing, snow, general	413	493	604
Skiing, water	354	422	518
Ski-mobiling, water	413	493	604
Skin diving, scuba diving, general	413	493	604
Sledding, tobogganing, bobsledding, luge	413	493	604
Snorkeling	295	352	431
Snowshoeing	472	563	690
Snowmobiling	207	246	302
Soccer, casual, general	413	493	604
Soccer, competitive	590	704	863
Softball or baseball, fast or slow pitch	295	352	431
Softball, officiating	354	422	518
Squash	708	844	1,035
Stair-treadmill ergometer, general	354	422	518
Standing-packing/unpacking boxes	207	246	302
Stretching, hatha yoga	236	281	345
Surfing, body or board	177	211	259
Sweeping garage, sidewalk	236	281	345
Swimming laps, freestyle, fast, vigorous effort	590	704	863
Swimming laps, freestyle, light/moderate effort	472	563	690
Swimming, backstroke, general	472	563	690
Swimming, breaststroke, general	590	704	863
Swimming, butterfly, general	649	774	949
Swimming, leisurely, general	354	422	518
Swimming, sidestroke, general	472	563	690
Swimming, synchronized	472	563	690
Swimming, treading water, fast/vigorous	590	704	863
Swimming, treading water, moderate effort	236	281	345

	130 LBS.	155 LBS.	190 LBS.
Table tennis, ping pong	236	281	345
Tai chi	236	281	345
Teaching aerobics class	354	422	518
Tennis, doubles	354	422	518
Tennis, general	413	493	604
Tennis, singles	472	563	690
Unicycling	295	352	431
Volleyball, beach	472	563	690
Volleyball, competitive, in gymnasium	236	281	345
Volleyball, noncompetitive; 6 to 9 member team	177	211	259
Walk/run-playing with children-moderate	236	281	345
Walk/run-playing with children-vigorous	295	352	431
Walking, 2 mph, slow pace	148	176	216
Walking, 3 mph, moderate pace, walking dog	207	246	302
Walking, 3.5 mph, uphill	354	422	518
Walking, 4 mph, very brisk pace	236	281	345
Walking, carrying infant or 15-lb. load	207	246	302
Walking, grass track	295	352	431
Walking, upstairs	472	563	690
Walking, using crutches	236	281	345
Wallyball, general	413	493	604
Water aerobics, water calisthenics	236	281	345
Water polo	590	704	863
Water volleyball	177	211	259
Weight lifting or body building, vigorous effort	354	422	518
Weight lifting, light or moderate effort	177	211	259
Whitewater rafting, kayaking, or canoeing	295	352	431

GOALS

Here is where your journal begins. List your goals, and not just the numbers! Write down how you expect to look and feel after 90 days. Write down all the reasons you are starting a healthier lifestyle. Write down all the positive things you want to have happen as a result of a new and improved you!

WEIGHT

Healthy weight loss averages about two pounds per week. You may see more rapid results than this in the beginning, especially if you are more than 50 pounds overweight. To lose weight the right way and keep it off, you may not reach your **OVERALL GOAL WEIGHT** in 90 days, but you will make huge strides towards it. Pick a **90-DAY GOAL WEIGHT** that is healthy *and* realistic.

90-DAY GOAL WEIGHT _____

Using the BMI chart, determine your Overall Goal Weight.

OVERALL GOAL WEIGHT _____

CALORIES

To find the right **DAILY CALORIE BALANCE** for you, use this following formula:

Your weight x 15 (calories to maintain current weight) = current average calorie intake

Current average calorie intake – 500 = 1 lb. lost per week

Current average calorie intake – 750 = 1 – 1½ lb. lost per week

Current average calorie intake – 1000 = 2 lbs. lost per week

DAILY CALORIE BALANCE _____

Each week you will recalculate your **DAILY CALORIE BALANCE** based on your new weight.

Remember, women should eat at least 1,200 calories per day and men should eat 1,500 to maintain a healthy diet.

FAT

Diet experts recommend consuming between 20% and 30% of your daily calories through fat. Each gram of fat contains nine calories, so if you figure out that you should be on a diet of 1,500 calories per day, then you should eat between 33 and 50 grams of fat per day.

To find the right **DAILY FAT BALANCE** for you, use this following formula:

DAILY CALORIE BALANCE x .25 (healthy percent of fat of calories from fat) ÷ 9 (calories in a gram of fat) = **DAILY FAT BALANCE** (in grams)

DAILY FAT BALANCE _____

Each week you will recalculate your Daily Fat Balance based on your new weight.

OVERALL GOALS

USING YOUR JOURNAL

Your journal will be your quick-reference, easy-to-use, all-inclusive tracker. Use it to record the protein, carbs, fat, and calories in all the foods you eat. Keeping records will show you which foods are your favorites, which you find hard to resist, what you need to cut from or add to your diet, and hold you accountable for everything you eat.

In addition to your diet, you will record all the exercise that you do and how many calories you burned doing it. You will also be tracking how much water you drink. Plus, there is a Comments section where you can write down whatever you want for that day: where you went right or wrong, recipes or foods you come across that you love and love you back, or something that inspired you to stay the course.

Every 7 days, and then on the 90th day, you will remind yourself of your **90-DAY GOAL WEIGHT** and record your current weight, how much weight you've lost or gained, and how many pounds you have left to go to reach your **90-DAY GOAL WEIGHT**. Watching your progress will be a great reminder of how well you're doing, or what you still need to change.

The next two pages are from a sample journal. This sample dieter is a 5' 6" woman who started out at 182 pounds. This week she's calculating her daily calorie and fat balances by her new weight of 172. Take a look at how she's doing. After that, you'll be fully prepared to start your new healthy, feel-better, look-better life.

CALORIE GOAL <u>1,580</u>   **FAT GOAL** <u>44</u>

FOOD

TIME	AMT.	FOOD	PROTEIN (G)	CARBS (G)	CAL.	CAL. BALANCE	FAT (G)	FAT BALANCE
7:30 A.M.	8 oz.	cranberry juice	-	34	144	1,436	-	
	1 cup	coffee w/1 sugar	-	4	20	1,416	-	
	2	eggs	12	-	132	1,284	8	36
1 P.M.	½	head of Boston lettuce	-	2	11	1,273	-	
	1	tomato	2	7	38	1,235	1	35
	¼ cup	shredded cheddar	7	-	113	1,122	9	26
	2 tbs.	low-cal blue cheese dressing	1	-	30	1,092	2	24
	12 oz.	diet soda	-	4	-		-	
3 P.M.	3	chocolate chip cookies	1	16	144	948	6	18
6 P.M.	½	chicken breast	27	-	142	806	3	15
	1 tbs.	olive oil	-	-	119	687	14	1
	1	baked potato	5	63	220	467	-	
	1 cup	string beans	2	10	44	423	-	-
	7 oz.	white wine	-	5	140	283	-	
7 P.M.	1 cup	vanilla ice cream	4	34	(236)	47	(14)	-4
			61	179		47		-64
		TOTALS FOR TODAY						

# of 8-ounce glasses of water drank today:

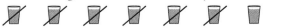

EXERCISE

STRETCHING / WARMING UP / FLEXIBILITY

TIME	TYPE	DURATION	CAL. BURNED	CLASS GROUP ACTIVITY
7 A.M.	yoga	½ hour	140	yes
10:55 A.M.	stretching	5 min	23	
5:15 P.M.	stretching	15 min	70	
		TOTAL	223	

STRENGTH TRAINING / WEIGHT LIFTING

TIME	TYPE	DURATION	CAL. BURNED	CLASS GROUP ACTIVITY
11 A.M.	lifting arm weights	15 min	105	
11:15 A.M.	sit-ups	15 min	139.5	
		TOTAL	144.5	

CARDIOVASCULAR

TIME	TYPE	DURATION	CAL. BURNED	CLASS GROUP ACTIVITY
5:30 P.M.	jogging	½ hour	246	
		TOTAL	246	

TOTAL CALORIES BURNED TODAY _613.5_

WEEKLY WEIGH-IN:

ORIGINAL WEIGHT _182_ **NEW WEIGHT** _170_ **WEIGHT CHANGE** _12_

POUNDS LEFT BEFORE MY 90-DAY GOAL IS REACHED _13_

RECALCULATED DAILY CALORIE BALANCE FOR NEXT WEEK _1,550_

RECALCULATED DAILY FAT BALANCE FOR NEXT WEEK _43_

NOTES ABOUT THIS WEEK: _I can't believe I'm already almost halfway there! I can fit back into that dress I bought for Ali's wedding 3 years ago—I just had to try it on again. Next week is going to be tough since I'm going out to dinner with clients, but that just means I'll have to stay on the exercise bike. And no more ice cream!_

DATE 30 Nov. 2010   **DAY 1**

CALORIE GOAL _____   FAT GOAL _____

FOOD

TIME	AMT.	FOOD	PROTEIN (G)	CARBS (G)	CAL.	CAL. BALANCE	FAT (G)	FAT BALANCE
		TOTALS FOR TODAY						

# of 8-ounce glasses of water drank today:

Fat 23.7% BMI 20.4   129.5 lbs

EXERCISE

STRETCHING / WARMING UP / FLEXIBILITY

TIME	TYPE	DURATION	CAL. BURNED	CLASS GROUP ACTIVITY
	TOTAL			

STRENGTH TRAINING / WEIGHT LIFTING

TIME	TYPE	DURATION	CAL. BURNED	CLASS GROUP ACTIVITY
	TOTAL			

CARDIOVASCULAR

TIME	TYPE	DURATION	CAL. BURNED	CLASS GROUP ACTIVITY
9:30	Eliptricycle	45	350	
	TOTAL			

TOTAL CALORIES BURNED TODAY _____

COMMENTS ON TODAY'S FOOD AND EXERCISE/GOALS FOR TOMORROW:

_____

_____

_____

_____

_____

_____

_____

DATE   **DAY 2**

CALORIE GOAL _____   FAT GOAL _____

FOOD

TIME	AMT.	FOOD	PROTEIN (G)	CARBS (G)	CAL.	CAL. BALANCE	FAT (G)	FAT BALANCE
		TOTALS FOR TODAY						

# of 8-ounce glasses of water drank today:

EXERCISE

STRETCHING / WARMING UP / FLEXIBILITY

TIME	TYPE	DURATION	CAL. BURNED	CLASS GROUP ACTIVITY
		TOTAL		

STRENGTH TRAINING / WEIGHT LIFTING

TIME	TYPE	DURATION	CAL. BURNED	CLASS GROUP ACTIVITY
		TOTAL		

CARDIOVASCULAR

TIME	TYPE	DURATION	CAL. BURNED	CLASS GROUP ACTIVITY
		TOTAL		

TOTAL CALORIES BURNED TODAY _____

COMMENTS ON TODAY'S FOOD AND EXERCISE/GOALS FOR TOMORROW:

_____

_____

_____

_____

_____

_____

_____

DATE   **DAY 3**

CALORIE GOAL _____   FAT GOAL _____

FOOD

TIME	AMT.	FOOD	PROTEIN (G)	CARBS (G)	CAL.	CAL. BALANCE	FAT (G)	FAT BALANCE
		TOTALS FOR TODAY						

# of 8-ounce glasses of water drank today:

EXERCISE

STRETCHING / WARMING UP / FLEXIBILITY

TIME	TYPE	DURATION	CAL. BURNED	CLASS GROUP ACTIVITY
		TOTAL		

STRENGTH TRAINING / WEIGHT LIFTING

TIME	TYPE	DURATION	CAL. BURNED	CLASS GROUP ACTIVITY
		TOTAL		

CARDIOVASCULAR

TIME	TYPE	DURATION	CAL. BURNED	CLASS GROUP ACTIVITY
		TOTAL		

TOTAL CALORIES BURNED TODAY _____

COMMENTS ON TODAY'S FOOD AND EXERCISE/GOALS FOR TOMORROW:

_____

_____

_____

_____

_____

_____

_____

DATE

DAY 4

CALORIE GOAL _____   FAT GOAL _____

FOOD

TIME	AMT.	FOOD	PROTEIN (G)	CARBS (G)	CAL.	CAL. BALANCE	FAT (G)	FAT BALANCE
		TOTALS FOR TODAY						

# of 8-ounce glasses of water drank today:

EXERCISE

STRETCHING / WARMING UP / FLEXIBILITY

TIME	TYPE	DURATION	CAL. BURNED	CLASS GROUP ACTIVITY
		TOTAL		

STRENGTH TRAINING / WEIGHT LIFTING

TIME	TYPE	DURATION	CAL. BURNED	CLASS GROUP ACTIVITY
		TOTAL		

CARDIOVASCULAR

TIME	TYPE	DURATION	CAL. BURNED	CLASS GROUP ACTIVITY
		TOTAL		

TOTAL CALORIES BURNED TODAY _____

COMMENTS ON TODAY'S FOOD AND EXERCISE/GOALS FOR TOMORROW:

_____

_____

_____

_____

_____

_____

_____

DATE

DAY 5

CALORIE GOAL _____   FAT GOAL _____

FOOD

TIME	AMT.	FOOD	PROTEIN (G)	CARBS (G)	CAL.	CAL. BALANCE	FAT (G)	FAT BALANCE
		TOTALS FOR TODAY						

# of 8-ounce glasses of water drank today:

EXERCISE

STRETCHING / WARMING UP / FLEXIBILITY

TIME	TYPE	DURATION	CAL. BURNED	CLASS GROUP ACTIVITY
		TOTAL		

STRENGTH TRAINING / WEIGHT LIFTING

TIME	TYPE	DURATION	CAL. BURNED	CLASS GROUP ACTIVITY
		TOTAL		

CARDIOVASCULAR

TIME	TYPE	DURATION	CAL. BURNED	CLASS GROUP ACTIVITY
		TOTAL		

TOTAL CALORIES BURNED TODAY _____

COMMENTS ON TODAY'S FOOD AND EXERCISE/GOALS FOR TOMORROW:

_____

_____

_____

_____

_____

_____

_____

CALORIE GOAL _____   FAT GOAL _____

FOOD

TIME	AMT.	FOOD	PROTEIN (G)	CARBS (G)	CAL.	CAL. BALANCE	FAT (G)	FAT BALANCE
		TOTALS FOR TODAY						

# of 8-ounce glasses of water drank today:

EXERCISE

STRETCHING / WARMING UP / FLEXIBILITY

TIME	TYPE	DURATION	CAL. BURNED	CLASS GROUP ACTIVITY
		TOTAL		

STRENGTH TRAINING / WEIGHT LIFTING

TIME	TYPE	DURATION	CAL. BURNED	CLASS GROUP ACTIVITY
		TOTAL		

CARDIOVASCULAR

TIME	TYPE	DURATION	CAL. BURNED	CLASS GROUP ACTIVITY
		TOTAL		

TOTAL CALORIES BURNED TODAY _____

COMMENTS ON TODAY'S FOOD AND EXERCISE/GOALS FOR TOMORROW:

_____

_____

_____

_____

_____

_____

_____

CALORIE GOAL _____   **FAT GOAL** _____

FOOD

TIME	AMT.	FOOD	PROTEIN (G)	CARBS (G)	CAL.	CAL. BALANCE	FAT (G)	FAT BALANCE
		TOTALS FOR TODAY						

# of 8-ounce glasses of water drank today:

EXERCISE

STRETCHING / WARMING UP / FLEXIBILITY

TIME	TYPE	DURATION	CAL. BURNED	CLASS GROUP ACTIVITY
		TOTAL		

STRENGTH TRAINING / WEIGHT LIFTING

TIME	TYPE	DURATION	CAL. BURNED	CLASS GROUP ACTIVITY
		TOTAL		

CARDIOVASCULAR

TIME	TYPE	DURATION	CAL. BURNED	CLASS GROUP ACTIVITY
		TOTAL		

TOTAL CALORIES BURNED TODAY _____

WEEKLY WEIGH-IN:

ORIGINAL WEIGHT _____ NEW WEIGHT _____ WEIGHT CHANGE _____

POUNDS LEFT BEFORE MY 90-DAY GOAL IS REACHED _____

RECALCULATED DAILY CALORIE BALANCE FOR NEXT WEEK _____

RECALCULATED DAILY FAT BALANCE FOR NEXT WEEK _____

NOTES ABOUT THIS WEEK: _____

_____

_____

_____

DAY 8

CALORIE GOAL _____ **FAT GOAL** _____

FOOD

TIME	AMT.	FOOD	PROTEIN (G)	CARBS (G)	CAL.	CAL. BALANCE	FAT (G)	FAT BALANCE
		TOTALS FOR TODAY						

# of 8-ounce glasses of water drank today:

EXERCISE

STRETCHING / WARMING UP / FLEXIBILITY

TIME	TYPE	DURATION	CAL. BURNED	CLASS GROUP ACTIVITY
	TOTAL			

STRENGTH TRAINING / WEIGHT LIFTING

TIME	TYPE	DURATION	CAL. BURNED	CLASS GROUP ACTIVITY
	TOTAL			

CARDIOVASCULAR

TIME	TYPE	DURATION	CAL. BURNED	CLASS GROUP ACTIVITY
	TOTAL			

TOTAL CALORIES BURNED TODAY _____

COMMENTS ON TODAY'S FOOD AND EXERCISE/GOALS FOR TOMORROW:

_____

_____

_____

_____

_____

_____

_____

DATE   **DAY 9**

CALORIE GOAL _____   FAT GOAL _____

FOOD

TIME	AMT.	FOOD	PROTEIN (G)	CARBS (G)	CAL.	CAL. BALANCE	FAT (G)	FAT BALANCE
		TOTALS FOR TODAY						

# of 8-ounce glasses of water drank today:

EXERCISE

STRETCHING / WARMING UP / FLEXIBILITY

TIME	TYPE	DURATION	CAL. BURNED	CLASS GROUP ACTIVITY
	TOTAL			

STRENGTH TRAINING / WEIGHT LIFTING

TIME	TYPE	DURATION	CAL. BURNED	CLASS GROUP ACTIVITY
	TOTAL			

CARDIOVASCULAR

TIME	TYPE	DURATION	CAL. BURNED	CLASS GROUP ACTIVITY
	TOTAL			

TOTAL CALORIES BURNED TODAY _____

COMMENTS ON TODAY'S FOOD AND EXERCISE/GOALS FOR TOMORROW:

_____

_____

_____

_____

_____

_____

_____

_____

CALORIE GOAL _____   FAT GOAL _____

FOOD

TIME	AMT.	FOOD	PROTEIN (G)	CARBS (G)	CAL.	CAL. BALANCE	FAT (G)	FAT BALANCE
		TOTALS FOR TODAY						

# of 8-ounce glasses of water drank today:

EXERCISE

STRETCHING / WARMING UP / FLEXIBILITY

TIME	TYPE	DURATION	CAL. BURNED	CLASS GROUP ACTIVITY
		TOTAL		

STRENGTH TRAINING / WEIGHT LIFTING

TIME	TYPE	DURATION	CAL. BURNED	CLASS GROUP ACTIVITY
		TOTAL		

CARDIOVASCULAR

TIME	TYPE	DURATION	CAL. BURNED	CLASS GROUP ACTIVITY
		TOTAL		

TOTAL CALORIES BURNED TODAY _____

COMMENTS ON TODAY'S FOOD AND EXERCISE/GOALS FOR TOMORROW:

_____

_____

_____

_____

_____

_____

_____

DATE   **DAY 11**

CALORIE GOAL _____   FAT GOAL _____

FOOD

TIME	AMT.	FOOD	PROTEIN (G)	CARBS (G)	CAL.	CAL. BALANCE	FAT (G)	FAT BALANCE
		TOTALS FOR TODAY						

# of 8-ounce glasses of water drank today:

48

EXERCISE

STRETCHING / WARMING UP / FLEXIBILITY

TIME	TYPE	DURATION	CAL. BURNED	CLASS GROUP ACTIVITY
		TOTAL		

STRENGTH TRAINING / WEIGHT LIFTING

TIME	TYPE	DURATION	CAL. BURNED	CLASS GROUP ACTIVITY
		TOTAL		

CARDIOVASCULAR

TIME	TYPE	DURATION	CAL. BURNED	CLASS GROUP ACTIVITY
		TOTAL		

TOTAL CALORIES BURNED TODAY _____

COMMENTS ON TODAY'S FOOD AND EXERCISE/GOALS FOR TOMORROW:

_____

_____

_____

_____

_____

_____

_____

DATE   **DAY 12**

CALORIE GOAL _____   FAT GOAL _____

FOOD

TIME	AMT.	FOOD	PROTEIN (G)	CARBS (G)	CAL.	CAL. BALANCE	FAT (G)	FAT BALANCE
		TOTALS FOR TODAY						

# of 8-ounce glasses of water drank today:

EXERCISE

STRETCHING / WARMING UP / FLEXIBILITY

TIME	TYPE	DURATION	CAL. BURNED	CLASS GROUP ACTIVITY
		TOTAL		

STRENGTH TRAINING / WEIGHT LIFTING

TIME	TYPE	DURATION	CAL. BURNED	CLASS GROUP ACTIVITY
		TOTAL		

CARDIOVASCULAR

TIME	TYPE	DURATION	CAL. BURNED	CLASS GROUP ACTIVITY
		TOTAL		

TOTAL CALORIES BURNED TODAY _____

COMMENTS ON TODAY'S FOOD AND EXERCISE/GOALS FOR TOMORROW:

_____

_____

_____

_____

_____

_____

_____

DATE   DAY 13

CALORIE GOAL _____   FAT GOAL _____

FOOD

TIME	AMT.	FOOD	PROTEIN (G)	CARBS (G)	CAL.	CAL. BALANCE	FAT (G)	FAT BALANCE
		TOTALS FOR TODAY						

# of 8-ounce glasses of water drank today:

EXERCISE

STRETCHING / WARMING UP / FLEXIBILITY

TIME	TYPE	DURATION	CAL. BURNED	CLASS GROUP ACTIVITY
		TOTAL		

STRENGTH TRAINING / WEIGHT LIFTING

TIME	TYPE	DURATION	CAL. BURNED	CLASS GROUP ACTIVITY
		TOTAL		

CARDIOVASCULAR

TIME	TYPE	DURATION	CAL. BURNED	CLASS GROUP ACTIVITY
		TOTAL		

TOTAL CALORIES BURNED TODAY _____

COMMENTS ON TODAY'S FOOD AND EXERCISE/GOALS FOR TOMORROW:

_____

_____

_____

_____

_____

_____

_____

DATE   DAY 14

CALORIE GOAL _____   FAT GOAL _____

FOOD

TIME	AMT.	FOOD	PROTEIN (G)	CARBS (G)	CAL.	CAL. BALANCE	FAT (G)	FAT BALANCE
		TOTALS FOR TODAY						

# of 8-ounce glasses of water drank today:

EXERCISE

STRETCHING / WARMING UP / FLEXIBILITY

TIME	TYPE	DURATION	CAL. BURNED	CLASS GROUP ACTIVITY
	TOTAL			

STRENGTH TRAINING / WEIGHT LIFTING

TIME	TYPE	DURATION	CAL. BURNED	CLASS GROUP ACTIVITY
	TOTAL			

CARDIOVASCULAR

TIME	TYPE	DURATION	CAL. BURNED	CLASS GROUP ACTIVITY
	TOTAL			

TOTAL CALORIES BURNED TODAY _____

WEEKLY WEIGH-IN:

ORIGINAL WEIGHT _____ NEW WEIGHT _____ WEIGHT CHANGE _____

POUNDS LEFT BEFORE MY 90-DAY GOAL IS REACHED _____

RECALCULATED DAILY CALORIE BALANCE FOR NEXT WEEK _____

RECALCULATED DAILY FAT BALANCE FOR NEXT WEEK _____

NOTES ABOUT THIS WEEK: _____

_____

_____

_____

CALORIE GOAL _____   **FAT GOAL** _____

FOOD

TIME	AMT.	FOOD	PROTEIN (G)	CARBS (G)	CAL.	CAL. BALANCE	FAT (G)	FAT BALANCE
		TOTALS FOR TODAY						

# of 8-ounce glasses of water drank today:

EXERCISE

STRETCHING / WARMING UP / FLEXIBILITY

TIME	TYPE	DURATION	CAL. BURNED	CLASS GROUP ACTIVITY
	TOTAL			

STRENGTH TRAINING / WEIGHT LIFTING

TIME	TYPE	DURATION	CAL. BURNED	CLASS GROUP ACTIVITY
	TOTAL			

CARDIOVASCULAR

TIME	TYPE	DURATION	CAL. BURNED	CLASS GROUP ACTIVITY
	TOTAL			

TOTAL CALORIES BURNED TODAY _____

COMMENTS ON TODAY'S FOOD AND EXERCISE/GOALS FOR TOMORROW:

_____

_____

_____

_____

_____

_____

_____

_____

DATE

DAY 16

CALORIE GOAL _____   FAT GOAL _____

FOOD

TIME	AMT.	FOOD	PROTEIN (G)	CARBS (G)	CAL.	CAL. BALANCE	FAT (G)	FAT BALANCE
		TOTALS FOR TODAY						

# of 8-ounce glasses of water drank today:

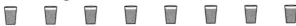

58

EXERCISE

STRETCHING / WARMING UP / FLEXIBILITY

TIME	TYPE	DURATION	CAL. BURNED	CLASS GROUP ACTIVITY
		TOTAL		

STRENGTH TRAINING / WEIGHT LIFTING

TIME	TYPE	DURATION	CAL. BURNED	CLASS GROUP ACTIVITY
		TOTAL		

CARDIOVASCULAR

TIME	TYPE	DURATION	CAL. BURNED	CLASS GROUP ACTIVITY
		TOTAL		

TOTAL CALORIES BURNED TODAY _____

COMMENTS ON TODAY'S FOOD AND EXERCISE/GOALS FOR TOMORROW:

_____

_____

_____

_____

_____

_____

_____

DAY 17

CALORIE GOAL _____   FAT GOAL _____

FOOD

TIME	AMT.	FOOD	PROTEIN (G)	CARBS (G)	CAL.	CAL. BALANCE	FAT (G)	FAT BALANCE
		TOTALS FOR TODAY						

# of 8-ounce glasses of water drank today:

EXERCISE

STRETCHING / WARMING UP / FLEXIBILITY

TIME	TYPE	DURATION	CAL. BURNED	CLASS GROUP ACTIVITY
		TOTAL		

STRENGTH TRAINING / WEIGHT LIFTING

TIME	TYPE	DURATION	CAL. BURNED	CLASS GROUP ACTIVITY
		TOTAL		

CARDIOVASCULAR

TIME	TYPE	DURATION	CAL. BURNED	CLASS GROUP ACTIVITY
		TOTAL		

TOTAL CALORIES BURNED TODAY _____

COMMENTS ON TODAY'S FOOD AND EXERCISE/GOALS FOR TOMORROW:

_____

_____

_____

_____

_____

_____

_____

_____

DAY 18

CALORIE GOAL _____   FAT GOAL _____

FOOD

TIME	AMT.	FOOD	PROTEIN (G)	CARBS (G)	CAL.	CAL. BALANCE	FAT (G)	FAT BALANCE
		TOTALS FOR TODAY						

# of 8-ounce glasses of water drank today:

EXERCISE

STRETCHING / WARMING UP / FLEXIBILITY

TIME	TYPE	DURATION	CAL. BURNED	CLASS GROUP ACTIVITY
		TOTAL		

STRENGTH TRAINING / WEIGHT LIFTING

TIME	TYPE	DURATION	CAL. BURNED	CLASS GROUP ACTIVITY
		TOTAL		

CARDIOVASCULAR

TIME	TYPE	DURATION	CAL. BURNED	CLASS GROUP ACTIVITY
		TOTAL		

TOTAL CALORIES BURNED TODAY _____

COMMENTS ON TODAY'S FOOD AND EXERCISE/GOALS FOR TOMORROW:

_____

_____

_____

_____

_____

_____

_____

_____

DATE   **DAY 19**

CALORIE GOAL _____   FAT GOAL _____

FOOD

TIME	AMT.	FOOD	PROTEIN (G)	CARBS (G)	CAL.	CAL. BALANCE	FAT (G)	FAT BALANCE
		TOTALS FOR TODAY						

\# of 8-ounce glasses of water drank today:

64

EXERCISE

STRETCHING / WARMING UP / FLEXIBILITY

TIME	TYPE	DURATION	CAL. BURNED	CLASS GROUP ACTIVITY
		TOTAL		

STRENGTH TRAINING / WEIGHT LIFTING

TIME	TYPE	DURATION	CAL. BURNED	CLASS GROUP ACTIVITY
		TOTAL		

CARDIOVASCULAR

TIME	TYPE	DURATION	CAL. BURNED	CLASS GROUP ACTIVITY
		TOTAL		

TOTAL CALORIES BURNED TODAY _____

COMMENTS ON TODAY'S FOOD AND EXERCISE/GOALS FOR TOMORROW:

_____

_____

_____

_____

_____

_____

_____

DAY 20

CALORIE GOAL _____ **FAT GOAL** _____

FOOD

TIME	AMT.	FOOD	PROTEIN (G)	CARBS (G)	CAL.	CAL. BALANCE	FAT (G)	FAT BALANCE
		TOTALS FOR TODAY						

# of 8-ounce glasses of water drank today:

EXERCISE

STRETCHING / WARMING UP / FLEXIBILITY

TIME	TYPE	DURATION	CAL. BURNED	CLASS GROUP ACTIVITY
		TOTAL		

STRENGTH TRAINING / WEIGHT LIFTING

TIME	TYPE	DURATION	CAL. BURNED	CLASS GROUP ACTIVITY
		TOTAL		

CARDIOVASCULAR

TIME	TYPE	DURATION	CAL. BURNED	CLASS GROUP ACTIVITY
		TOTAL		

TOTAL CALORIES BURNED TODAY _____

COMMENTS ON TODAY'S FOOD AND EXERCISE/GOALS FOR TOMORROW:

_____

_____

_____

_____

_____

_____

_____

_____

DAY 21

CALORIE GOAL _____   FAT GOAL _____

FOOD

TIME	AMT.	FOOD	PROTEIN (G)	CARBS (G)	CAL.	CAL. BALANCE	FAT (G)	FAT BALANCE
		TOTALS FOR TODAY						

# of 8-ounce glasses of water drank today:

EXERCISE

STRETCHING / WARMING UP / FLEXIBILITY

TIME	TYPE	DURATION	CAL. BURNED	CLASS GROUP ACTIVITY
		TOTAL		

STRENGTH TRAINING / WEIGHT LIFTING

TIME	TYPE	DURATION	CAL. BURNED	CLASS GROUP ACTIVITY
		TOTAL		

CARDIOVASCULAR

TIME	TYPE	DURATION	CAL. BURNED	CLASS GROUP ACTIVITY
		TOTAL		

TOTAL CALORIES BURNED TODAY _____

WEEKLY WEIGH-IN:

ORIGINAL WEIGHT _____ NEW WEIGHT _____ WEIGHT CHANGE _____

POUNDS LEFT BEFORE MY 90-DAY GOAL IS REACHED _____

RECALCULATED DAILY CALORIE BALANCE FOR NEXT WEEK _____

RECALCULATED DAILY FAT BALANCE FOR NEXT WEEK _____

NOTES ABOUT THIS WEEK: _____

_____

_____

_____

DATE

DAY 22

CALORIE GOAL _____   FAT GOAL _____

FOOD

TIME	AMT.	FOOD	PROTEIN (G)	CARBS (G)	CAL.	CAL. BALANCE	FAT (G)	FAT BALANCE
		TOTALS FOR TODAY						

# of 8-ounce glasses of water drank today:

EXERCISE

STRETCHING / WARMING UP / FLEXIBILITY

TIME	TYPE	DURATION	CAL. BURNED	CLASS GROUP ACTIVITY
	TOTAL			

STRENGTH TRAINING / WEIGHT LIFTING

TIME	TYPE	DURATION	CAL. BURNED	CLASS GROUP ACTIVITY
	TOTAL			

CARDIOVASCULAR

TIME	TYPE	DURATION	CAL. BURNED	CLASS GROUP ACTIVITY
	TOTAL			

TOTAL CALORIES BURNED TODAY _____

COMMENTS ON TODAY'S FOOD AND EXERCISE/GOALS FOR TOMORROW:

_____

_____

_____

_____

_____

_____

_____

_____

DAY 23

CALORIE GOAL _____   FAT GOAL _____

FOOD

TIME	AMT.	FOOD	PROTEIN (G)	CARBS (G)	CAL.	CAL. BALANCE	FAT (G)	FAT BALANCE
		TOTALS FOR TODAY						

# of 8-ounce glasses of water drank today:

EXERCISE

STRETCHING / WARMING UP / FLEXIBILITY

TIME	TYPE	DURATION	CAL. BURNED	CLASS GROUP ACTIVITY
		TOTAL		

STRENGTH TRAINING / WEIGHT LIFTING

TIME	TYPE	DURATION	CAL. BURNED	CLASS GROUP ACTIVITY
		TOTAL		

CARDIOVASCULAR

TIME	TYPE	DURATION	CAL. BURNED	CLASS GROUP ACTIVITY
		TOTAL		

TOTAL CALORIES BURNED TODAY _____

COMMENTS ON TODAY'S FOOD AND EXERCISE/GOALS FOR TOMORROW:

_____

_____

_____

_____

_____

_____

_____

_____

CALORIE GOAL _____   FAT GOAL _____

FOOD

TIME	AMT.	FOOD	PROTEIN (G)	CARBS (G)	CAL.	CAL. BALANCE	FAT (G)	FAT BALANCE
		TOTALS FOR TODAY						

# of 8-ounce glasses of water drank today:

EXERCISE

STRETCHING / WARMING UP / FLEXIBILITY

TIME	TYPE	DURATION	CAL. BURNED	CLASS GROUP ACTIVITY
		TOTAL		

STRENGTH TRAINING / WEIGHT LIFTING

TIME	TYPE	DURATION	CAL. BURNED	CLASS GROUP ACTIVITY
		TOTAL		

CARDIOVASCULAR

TIME	TYPE	DURATION	CAL. BURNED	CLASS GROUP ACTIVITY
		TOTAL		

TOTAL CALORIES BURNED TODAY _____

COMMENTS ON TODAY'S FOOD AND EXERCISE/GOALS FOR TOMORROW:

_____

_____

_____

_____

_____

_____

_____

_____

CALORIE GOAL _____   FAT GOAL _____

FOOD

TIME	AMT.	FOOD	PROTEIN (G)	CARBS (G)	CAL.	CAL. BALANCE	FAT (G)	FAT BALANCE
		TOTALS FOR TODAY						

# of 8-ounce glasses of water drank today:

EXERCISE

STRETCHING / WARMING UP / FLEXIBILITY

TIME	TYPE	DURATION	CAL. BURNED	CLASS GROUP ACTIVITY
	TOTAL			

STRENGTH TRAINING / WEIGHT LIFTING

TIME	TYPE	DURATION	CAL. BURNED	CLASS GROUP ACTIVITY
	TOTAL			

CARDIOVASCULAR

TIME	TYPE	DURATION	CAL. BURNED	CLASS GROUP ACTIVITY
	TOTAL			

TOTAL CALORIES BURNED TODAY _____

COMMENTS ON TODAY'S FOOD AND EXERCISE/GOALS FOR TOMORROW:

_____

_____

_____

_____

_____

_____

_____

_____

CALORIE GOAL _____   FAT GOAL _____

FOOD

TIME	AMT.	FOOD	PROTEIN (G)	CARBS (G)	CAL.	CAL. BALANCE	FAT (G)	FAT BALANCE
		TOTALS FOR TODAY						

# of 8-ounce glasses of water drank today:

EXERCISE

STRETCHING / WARMING UP / FLEXIBILITY

TIME	TYPE	DURATION	CAL. BURNED	CLASS GROUP ACTIVITY
		TOTAL		

STRENGTH TRAINING / WEIGHT LIFTING

TIME	TYPE	DURATION	CAL. BURNED	CLASS GROUP ACTIVITY
		TOTAL		

CARDIOVASCULAR

TIME	TYPE	DURATION	CAL. BURNED	CLASS GROUP ACTIVITY
		TOTAL		

TOTAL CALORIES BURNED TODAY _____

COMMENTS ON TODAY'S FOOD AND EXERCISE/GOALS FOR TOMORROW:

_____

_____

_____

_____

_____

_____

_____

DATE

DAY 27

CALORIE GOAL _____   FAT GOAL _____

FOOD

TIME	AMT.	FOOD	PROTEIN (G)	CARBS (G)	CAL.	CAL. BALANCE	FAT (G)	FAT BALANCE
		TOTALS FOR TODAY						

# of 8-ounce glasses of water drank today:

EXERCISE

STRETCHING / WARMING UP / FLEXIBILITY

TIME	TYPE	DURATION	CAL. BURNED	CLASS GROUP ACTIVITY
		TOTAL		

STRENGTH TRAINING / WEIGHT LIFTING

TIME	TYPE	DURATION	CAL. BURNED	CLASS GROUP ACTIVITY
		TOTAL		

CARDIOVASCULAR

TIME	TYPE	DURATION	CAL. BURNED	CLASS GROUP ACTIVITY
		TOTAL		

TOTAL CALORIES BURNED TODAY _____

COMMENTS ON TODAY'S FOOD AND EXERCISE/GOALS FOR TOMORROW:

_____

_____

_____

_____

_____

_____

_____

CALORIE GOAL _____   FAT GOAL _____

FOOD

TIME	AMT.	FOOD	PROTEIN (G)	CARBS (G)	CAL.	CAL. BALANCE	FAT (G)	FAT BALANCE
		TOTALS FOR TODAY						

# of 8-ounce glasses of water drank today:

EXERCISE

STRETCHING / WARMING UP / FLEXIBILITY

TIME	TYPE	DURATION	CAL. BURNED	CLASS GROUP ACTIVITY
		TOTAL		

STRENGTH TRAINING / WEIGHT LIFTING

TIME	TYPE	DURATION	CAL. BURNED	CLASS GROUP ACTIVITY
		TOTAL		

CARDIOVASCULAR

TIME	TYPE	DURATION	CAL. BURNED	CLASS GROUP ACTIVITY
		TOTAL		

TOTAL CALORIES BURNED TODAY _____

WEEKLY WEIGH-IN:

ORIGINAL WEIGHT _____ NEW WEIGHT _____ WEIGHT CHANGE _____

POUNDS LEFT BEFORE MY 90-DAY GOAL IS REACHED _____

RECALCULATED DAILY CALORIE BALANCE FOR NEXT WEEK _____

RECALCULATED DAILY FAT BALANCE FOR NEXT WEEK _____

NOTES ABOUT THIS WEEK: _____

_____

_____

_____

DAY 29

CALORIE GOAL _____   **FAT GOAL** _____

FOOD

TIME	AMT.	FOOD	PROTEIN (G)	CARBS (G)	CAL.	CAL. BALANCE	FAT (G)	FAT BALANCE
		TOTALS FOR TODAY						

# of 8-ounce glasses of water drank today:

EXERCISE

STRETCHING / WARMING UP / FLEXIBILITY

TIME	TYPE	DURATION	CAL. BURNED	CLASS GROUP ACTIVITY
		TOTAL		

STRENGTH TRAINING / WEIGHT LIFTING

TIME	TYPE	DURATION	CAL. BURNED	CLASS GROUP ACTIVITY
		TOTAL		

CARDIOVASCULAR

TIME	TYPE	DURATION	CAL. BURNED	CLASS GROUP ACTIVITY
		TOTAL		

TOTAL CALORIES BURNED TODAY _____

COMMENTS ON TODAY'S FOOD AND EXERCISE/GOALS FOR TOMORROW:

_____

_____

_____

_____

_____

_____

_____

_____

DATE   DAY 30

CALORIE GOAL _____   FAT GOAL _____

FOOD

TIME	AMT.	FOOD	PROTEIN (G)	CARBS (G)	CAL.	CAL. BALANCE	FAT (G)	FAT BALANCE
		TOTALS FOR TODAY						

# of 8-ounce glasses of water drank today:

EXERCISE

STRETCHING / WARMING UP / FLEXIBILITY

TIME	TYPE	DURATION	CAL. BURNED	CLASS GROUP ACTIVITY
		TOTAL		

STRENGTH TRAINING / WEIGHT LIFTING

TIME	TYPE	DURATION	CAL. BURNED	CLASS GROUP ACTIVITY
		TOTAL		

CARDIOVASCULAR

TIME	TYPE	DURATION	CAL. BURNED	CLASS GROUP ACTIVITY
		TOTAL		

TOTAL CALORIES BURNED TODAY _____

COMMENTS ON TODAY'S FOOD AND EXERCISE/GOALS FOR TOMORROW:

_____

_____

_____

_____

_____

_____

_____

_____

DATE

DAY 31

CALORIE GOAL _____   **FAT GOAL** _____

FOOD

TIME	AMT.	FOOD	PROTEIN (G)	CARBS (G)	CAL.	CAL. BALANCE	FAT (G)	FAT BALANCE
		TOTALS FOR TODAY						

# of 8-ounce glasses of water drank today:

EXERCISE

STRETCHING / WARMING UP / FLEXIBILITY

TIME	TYPE	DURATION	CAL. BURNED	CLASS GROUP ACTIVITY
		TOTAL		

STRENGTH TRAINING / WEIGHT LIFTING

TIME	TYPE	DURATION	CAL. BURNED	CLASS GROUP ACTIVITY
		TOTAL		

CARDIOVASCULAR

TIME	TYPE	DURATION	CAL. BURNED	CLASS GROUP ACTIVITY
		TOTAL		

TOTAL CALORIES BURNED TODAY _____

COMMENTS ON TODAY'S FOOD AND EXERCISE/GOALS FOR TOMORROW:

_____

_____

_____

_____

_____

_____

_____

_____

DAY 32

CALORIE GOAL _____   FAT GOAL _____

FOOD

TIME	AMT.	FOOD	PROTEIN (G)	CARBS (G)	CAL.	CAL. BALANCE	FAT (G)	FAT BALANCE
		TOTALS FOR TODAY						

# of 8-ounce glasses of water drank today:

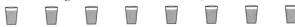

EXERCISE

STRETCHING / WARMING UP / FLEXIBILITY

TIME	TYPE	DURATION	CAL. BURNED	CLASS GROUP ACTIVITY
		TOTAL		

STRENGTH TRAINING / WEIGHT LIFTING

TIME	TYPE	DURATION	CAL. BURNED	CLASS GROUP ACTIVITY
		TOTAL		

CARDIOVASCULAR

TIME	TYPE	DURATION	CAL. BURNED	CLASS GROUP ACTIVITY
		TOTAL		

TOTAL CALORIES BURNED TODAY _____

COMMENTS ON TODAY'S FOOD AND EXERCISE/GOALS FOR TOMORROW:

_____

_____

_____

_____

_____

_____

_____

_____

CALORIE GOAL _____   FAT GOAL _____

FOOD

TIME	AMT.	FOOD	PROTEIN (G)	CARBS (G)	CAL.	CAL. BALANCE	FAT (G)	FAT BALANCE
		TOTALS FOR TODAY						

# of 8-ounce glasses of water drank today:

EXERCISE

STRETCHING / WARMING UP / FLEXIBILITY

TIME	TYPE	DURATION	CAL. BURNED	CLASS GROUP ACTIVITY
		TOTAL		

STRENGTH TRAINING / WEIGHT LIFTING

TIME	TYPE	DURATION	CAL. BURNED	CLASS GROUP ACTIVITY
		TOTAL		

CARDIOVASCULAR

TIME	TYPE	DURATION	CAL. BURNED	CLASS GROUP ACTIVITY
		TOTAL		

TOTAL CALORIES BURNED TODAY _____

COMMENTS ON TODAY'S FOOD AND EXERCISE/GOALS FOR TOMORROW:

_____

_____

_____

_____

_____

_____

_____

_____

DATE

DAY 34

CALORIE GOAL _____   FAT GOAL _____

FOOD

TIME	AMT.	FOOD	PROTEIN (G)	CARBS (G)	CAL.	CAL. BALANCE	FAT (G)	FAT BALANCE
		TOTALS FOR TODAY						

# of 8-ounce glasses of water drank today:

EXERCISE

STRETCHING / WARMING UP / FLEXIBILITY

TIME	TYPE	DURATION	CAL. BURNED	CLASS GROUP ACTIVITY
		TOTAL		

STRENGTH TRAINING / WEIGHT LIFTING

TIME	TYPE	DURATION	CAL. BURNED	CLASS GROUP ACTIVITY
		TOTAL		

CARDIOVASCULAR

TIME	TYPE	DURATION	CAL. BURNED	CLASS GROUP ACTIVITY
		TOTAL		

TOTAL CALORIES BURNED TODAY _____

COMMENTS ON TODAY'S FOOD AND EXERCISE/GOALS FOR TOMORROW:

_____

_____

_____

_____

_____

_____

_____

DAY 35

CALORIE GOAL _____   FAT GOAL _____

FOOD

TIME	AMT.	FOOD	PROTEIN (G)	CARBS (G)	CAL.	CAL. BALANCE	FAT (G)	FAT BALANCE
		TOTALS FOR TODAY						

# of 8-ounce glasses of water drank today:

EXERCISE

STRETCHING / WARMING UP / FLEXIBILITY

TIME	TYPE	DURATION	CAL. BURNED	CLASS GROUP ACTIVITY
		TOTAL		

STRENGTH TRAINING / WEIGHT LIFTING

TIME	TYPE	DURATION	CAL. BURNED	CLASS GROUP ACTIVITY
		TOTAL		

CARDIOVASCULAR

TIME	TYPE	DURATION	CAL. BURNED	CLASS GROUP ACTIVITY
		TOTAL		

TOTAL CALORIES BURNED TODAY _____

WEEKLY WEIGH-IN:

ORIGINAL WEIGHT _____ NEW WEIGHT _____ WEIGHT CHANGE _____

POUNDS LEFT BEFORE MY 90-DAY GOAL IS REACHED _____

RECALCULATED DAILY CALORIE BALANCE FOR NEXT WEEK _____

RECALCULATED DAILY FAT BALANCE FOR NEXT WEEK _____

NOTES ABOUT THIS WEEK: _____

_____

_____

_____

DAY 36

CALORIE GOAL _____   **FAT GOAL** _____

FOOD

TIME	AMT.	FOOD	PROTEIN (G)	CARBS (G)	CAL.	CAL. BALANCE	FAT (G)	FAT BALANCE
		TOTALS FOR TODAY						

# of 8-ounce glasses of water drank today:

EXERCISE

STRETCHING / WARMING UP / FLEXIBILITY

TIME	TYPE	DURATION	CAL. BURNED	CLASS GROUP ACTIVITY
		TOTAL		

STRENGTH TRAINING / WEIGHT LIFTING

TIME	TYPE	DURATION	CAL. BURNED	CLASS GROUP ACTIVITY
		TOTAL		

CARDIOVASCULAR

TIME	TYPE	DURATION	CAL. BURNED	CLASS GROUP ACTIVITY
		TOTAL		

TOTAL CALORIES BURNED TODAY _____

COMMENTS ON TODAY'S FOOD AND EXERCISE/GOALS FOR TOMORROW:

_____

_____

_____

_____

_____

_____

_____

DATE **DAY 37**

CALORIE GOAL _____   FAT GOAL _____

FOOD

TIME	AMT.	FOOD	PROTEIN (G)	CARBS (G)	CAL.	CAL. BALANCE	FAT (G)	FAT BALANCE
		TOTALS FOR TODAY						

# of 8-ounce glasses of water drank today:

EXERCISE

STRETCHING / WARMING UP / FLEXIBILITY

TIME	TYPE	DURATION	CAL. BURNED	CLASS GROUP ACTIVITY
	TOTAL			

STRENGTH TRAINING / WEIGHT LIFTING

TIME	TYPE	DURATION	CAL. BURNED	CLASS GROUP ACTIVITY
	TOTAL			

CARDIOVASCULAR

TIME	TYPE	DURATION	CAL. BURNED	CLASS GROUP ACTIVITY
	TOTAL			

TOTAL CALORIES BURNED TODAY _____

COMMENTS ON TODAY'S FOOD AND EXERCISE/GOALS FOR TOMORROW:

_____

_____

_____

_____

_____

_____

_____

_____

DATE

DAY 38

CALORIE GOAL _____   FAT GOAL _____

FOOD

TIME	AMT.	FOOD	PROTEIN (G)	CARBS (G)	CAL.	CAL. BALANCE	FAT (G)	FAT BALANCE
		TOTALS FOR TODAY						

# of 8-ounce glasses of water drank today:

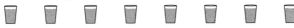

EXERCISE

STRETCHING / WARMING UP / FLEXIBILITY

TIME	TYPE	DURATION	CAL. BURNED	CLASS GROUP ACTIVITY
		TOTAL		

STRENGTH TRAINING / WEIGHT LIFTING

TIME	TYPE	DURATION	CAL. BURNED	CLASS GROUP ACTIVITY
		TOTAL		

CARDIOVASCULAR

TIME	TYPE	DURATION	CAL. BURNED	CLASS GROUP ACTIVITY
		TOTAL		

TOTAL CALORIES BURNED TODAY _____

COMMENTS ON TODAY'S FOOD AND EXERCISE/GOALS FOR TOMORROW:

_____

_____

_____

_____

_____

_____

_____

_____

DATE

DAY 39

CALORIE GOAL _____   FAT GOAL _____

FOOD

TIME	AMT.	FOOD	PROTEIN (G)	CARBS (G)	CAL.	CAL. BALANCE	FAT (G)	FAT BALANCE
		TOTALS FOR TODAY						

# of 8-ounce glasses of water drank today:

EXERCISE

STRETCHING / WARMING UP / FLEXIBILITY

TIME	TYPE	DURATION	CAL. BURNED	CLASS GROUP ACTIVITY
		TOTAL		

STRENGTH TRAINING / WEIGHT LIFTING

TIME	TYPE	DURATION	CAL. BURNED	CLASS GROUP ACTIVITY
		TOTAL		

CARDIOVASCULAR

TIME	TYPE	DURATION	CAL. BURNED	CLASS GROUP ACTIVITY
		TOTAL		

TOTAL CALORIES BURNED TODAY _____

COMMENTS ON TODAY'S FOOD AND EXERCISE/GOALS FOR TOMORROW:

_____

_____

_____

_____

_____

_____

_____

DAY 40

CALORIE GOAL _____ FAT GOAL _____

FOOD

TIME	AMT.	FOOD	PROTEIN (G)	CARBS (G)	CAL.	CAL. BALANCE	FAT (G)	FAT BALANCE
		TOTALS FOR TODAY						

# of 8-ounce glasses of water drank today:

EXERCISE

STRETCHING / WARMING UP / FLEXIBILITY

TIME	TYPE	DURATION	CAL. BURNED	CLASS GROUP ACTIVITY
		TOTAL		

STRENGTH TRAINING / WEIGHT LIFTING

TIME	TYPE	DURATION	CAL. BURNED	CLASS GROUP ACTIVITY
		TOTAL		

CARDIOVASCULAR

TIME	TYPE	DURATION	CAL. BURNED	CLASS GROUP ACTIVITY
		TOTAL		

TOTAL CALORIES BURNED TODAY _____

COMMENTS ON TODAY'S FOOD AND EXERCISE/GOALS FOR TOMORROW:

DATE **DAY 41**

CALORIE GOAL _____ FAT GOAL _____

FOOD

TIME	AMT.	FOOD	PROTEIN (G)	CARBS (G)	CAL.	CAL. BALANCE	FAT (G)	FAT BALANCE
	TOTALS FOR TODAY							

# of 8-ounce glasses of water drank today:

EXERCISE

STRETCHING / WARMING UP / FLEXIBILITY

TIME	TYPE	DURATION	CAL. BURNED	CLASS GROUP ACTIVITY
		TOTAL		

STRENGTH TRAINING / WEIGHT LIFTING

TIME	TYPE	DURATION	CAL. BURNED	CLASS GROUP ACTIVITY
		TOTAL		

CARDIOVASCULAR

TIME	TYPE	DURATION	CAL. BURNED	CLASS GROUP ACTIVITY
		TOTAL		

TOTAL CALORIES BURNED TODAY _____

COMMENTS ON TODAY'S FOOD AND EXERCISE/GOALS FOR TOMORROW:

_____

_____

_____

_____

_____

_____

_____

_____

DAY 42

CALORIE GOAL _____   FAT GOAL _____

FOOD

TIME	AMT.	FOOD	PROTEIN (G)	CARBS (G)	CAL.	CAL. BALANCE	FAT (G)	FAT BALANCE
	TOTALS FOR TODAY							

# of 8-ounce glasses of water drank today:

EXERCISE

STRETCHING / WARMING UP / FLEXIBILITY

TIME	TYPE	DURATION	CAL. BURNED	CLASS GROUP ACTIVITY
		TOTAL		

STRENGTH TRAINING / WEIGHT LIFTING

TIME	TYPE	DURATION	CAL. BURNED	CLASS GROUP ACTIVITY
		TOTAL		

CARDIOVASCULAR

TIME	TYPE	DURATION	CAL. BURNED	CLASS GROUP ACTIVITY
		TOTAL		

TOTAL CALORIES BURNED TODAY _____

WEEKLY WEIGH-IN:

ORIGINAL WEIGHT _____ **NEW WEIGHT** _____ **WEIGHT CHANGE** _____

POUNDS LEFT BEFORE MY 90-DAY GOAL IS REACHED _____

RECALCULATED DAILY CALORIE BALANCE FOR NEXT WEEK _____

RECALCULATED DAILY FAT BALANCE FOR NEXT WEEK _____

NOTES ABOUT THIS WEEK: _____

_____

_____

_____

CALORIE GOAL _____   FAT GOAL _____

FOOD

TIME	AMT.	FOOD	PROTEIN (G)	CARBS (G)	CAL.	CAL. BALANCE	FAT (G)	FAT BALANCE
		TOTALS FOR TODAY						

# of 8-ounce glasses of water drank today:

EXERCISE

STRETCHING / WARMING UP / FLEXIBILITY

TIME	TYPE	DURATION	CAL. BURNED	CLASS GROUP ACTIVITY
		TOTAL		

STRENGTH TRAINING / WEIGHT LIFTING

TIME	TYPE	DURATION	CAL. BURNED	CLASS GROUP ACTIVITY
		TOTAL		

CARDIOVASCULAR

TIME	TYPE	DURATION	CAL. BURNED	CLASS GROUP ACTIVITY
		TOTAL		

TOTAL CALORIES BURNED TODAY _____

COMMENTS ON TODAY'S FOOD AND EXERCISE/GOALS FOR TOMORROW:

_____

_____

_____

_____

_____

_____

_____

DAY 44

CALORIE GOAL _____   **FAT GOAL** _____

FOOD

TIME	AMT.	FOOD	PROTEIN (G)	CARBS (G)	CAL.	CAL. BALANCE	FAT (G)	FAT BALANCE
		TOTALS FOR TODAY						

# of 8-ounce glasses of water drank today:

EXERCISE

STRETCHING / WARMING UP / FLEXIBILITY

TIME	TYPE	DURATION	CAL. BURNED	CLASS GROUP ACTIVITY
		TOTAL		

STRENGTH TRAINING / WEIGHT LIFTING

TIME	TYPE	DURATION	CAL. BURNED	CLASS GROUP ACTIVITY
		TOTAL		

CARDIOVASCULAR

TIME	TYPE	DURATION	CAL. BURNED	CLASS GROUP ACTIVITY
		TOTAL		

TOTAL CALORIES BURNED TODAY _____

COMMENTS ON TODAY'S FOOD AND EXERCISE/GOALS FOR TOMORROW:

_____

_____

_____

_____

_____

_____

_____

DAY 45

CALORIE GOAL _____   FAT GOAL _____

FOOD

TIME	AMT.	FOOD	PROTEIN (G)	CARBS (G)	CAL.	CAL. BALANCE	FAT (G)	FAT BALANCE
		TOTALS FOR TODAY						

# of 8-ounce glasses of water drank today:

EXERCISE

STRETCHING / WARMING UP / FLEXIBILITY

TIME	TYPE	DURATION	CAL. BURNED	CLASS GROUP ACTIVITY
	TOTAL			

STRENGTH TRAINING / WEIGHT LIFTING

TIME	TYPE	DURATION	CAL. BURNED	CLASS GROUP ACTIVITY
	TOTAL			

CARDIOVASCULAR

TIME	TYPE	DURATION	CAL. BURNED	CLASS GROUP ACTIVITY
	TOTAL			

TOTAL CALORIES BURNED TODAY _____

COMMENTS ON TODAY'S FOOD AND EXERCISE/GOALS FOR TOMORROW:

_____

_____

_____

_____

_____

_____

_____

_____

DATE   DAY 46

CALORIE GOAL _____   FAT GOAL _____

FOOD

TIME	AMT.	FOOD	PROTEIN (G)	CARBS (G)	CAL.	CAL. BALANCE	FAT (G)	FAT BALANCE
		TOTALS FOR TODAY						

# of 8-ounce glasses of water drank today:

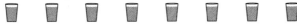

EXERCISE

STRETCHING / WARMING UP / FLEXIBILITY

TIME	TYPE	DURATION	CAL. BURNED	CLASS GROUP ACTIVITY
		TOTAL		

STRENGTH TRAINING / WEIGHT LIFTING

TIME	TYPE	DURATION	CAL. BURNED	CLASS GROUP ACTIVITY
		TOTAL		

CARDIOVASCULAR

TIME	TYPE	DURATION	CAL. BURNED	CLASS GROUP ACTIVITY
		TOTAL		

TOTAL CALORIES BURNED TODAY _____

COMMENTS ON TODAY'S FOOD AND EXERCISE/GOALS FOR TOMORROW:

_____

_____

_____

_____

_____

_____

_____

DAY 47

CALORIE GOAL _____   FAT GOAL _____

FOOD

TIME	AMT.	FOOD	PROTEIN (G)	CARBS (G)	CAL.	CAL. BALANCE	FAT (G)	FAT BALANCE
		TOTALS FOR TODAY						

# of 8-ounce glasses of water drank today:

EXERCISE

STRETCHING / WARMING UP / FLEXIBILITY

TIME	TYPE	DURATION	CAL. BURNED	CLASS GROUP ACTIVITY
		TOTAL		

STRENGTH TRAINING / WEIGHT LIFTING

TIME	TYPE	DURATION	CAL. BURNED	CLASS GROUP ACTIVITY
		TOTAL		

CARDIOVASCULAR

TIME	TYPE	DURATION	CAL. BURNED	CLASS GROUP ACTIVITY
		TOTAL		

TOTAL CALORIES BURNED TODAY _____

COMMENTS ON TODAY'S FOOD AND EXERCISE/GOALS FOR TOMORROW:

_____

_____

_____

_____

_____

_____

_____

_____

CALORIE GOAL _____　　　FAT GOAL _____

FOOD

TIME	AMT.	FOOD	PROTEIN (G)	CARBS (G)	CAL.	CAL. BALANCE	FAT (G)	FAT BALANCE
			TOTALS FOR TODAY						

# of 8-ounce glasses of water drank today:

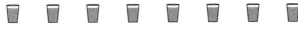

EXERCISE

STRETCHING / WARMING UP / FLEXIBILITY

TIME	TYPE	DURATION	CAL. BURNED	CLASS GROUP ACTIVITY
	TOTAL			

STRENGTH TRAINING / WEIGHT LIFTING

TIME	TYPE	DURATION	CAL. BURNED	CLASS GROUP ACTIVITY
	TOTAL			

CARDIOVASCULAR

TIME	TYPE	DURATION	CAL. BURNED	CLASS GROUP ACTIVITY
	TOTAL			

TOTAL CALORIES BURNED TODAY _____

COMMENTS ON TODAY'S FOOD AND EXERCISE/GOALS FOR TOMORROW:

_____

_____

_____

_____

_____

_____

_____

_____

123

DATE _____   **DAY 49**

CALORIE GOAL _____   FAT GOAL _____

FOOD

TIME	AMT.	FOOD	PROTEIN (G)	CARBS (G)	CAL.	CAL. BALANCE	FAT (G)	FAT BALANCE
		TOTALS FOR TODAY						

# of 8-ounce glasses of water drank today:

EXERCISE

STRETCHING / WARMING UP / FLEXIBILITY

TIME	TYPE	DURATION	CAL. BURNED	CLASS GROUP ACTIVITY
		TOTAL		

STRENGTH TRAINING / WEIGHT LIFTING

TIME	TYPE	DURATION	CAL. BURNED	CLASS GROUP ACTIVITY
		TOTAL		

CARDIOVASCULAR

TIME	TYPE	DURATION	CAL. BURNED	CLASS GROUP ACTIVITY
		TOTAL		

TOTAL CALORIES BURNED TODAY _____

WEEKLY WEIGH-IN:

ORIGINAL WEIGHT _____ NEW WEIGHT _____ WEIGHT CHANGE _____

POUNDS LEFT BEFORE MY 90-DAY GOAL IS REACHED _____

RECALCULATED DAILY CALORIE BALANCE FOR NEXT WEEK _____

RECALCULATED DAILY FAT BALANCE FOR NEXT WEEK _____

NOTES ABOUT THIS WEEK: _____

_____

_____

_____

DAY 50

CALORIE GOAL _____ FAT GOAL _____

FOOD

TIME	AMT.	FOOD	PROTEIN (G)	CARBS (G)	CAL.	CAL. BALANCE	FAT (G)	FAT BALANCE
		TOTALS FOR TODAY						

# of 8-ounce glasses of water drank today:

EXERCISE

STRETCHING / WARMING UP / FLEXIBILITY

TIME	TYPE	DURATION	CAL. BURNED	CLASS GROUP ACTIVITY
		TOTAL		

STRENGTH TRAINING / WEIGHT LIFTING

TIME	TYPE	DURATION	CAL. BURNED	CLASS GROUP ACTIVITY
		TOTAL		

CARDIOVASCULAR

TIME	TYPE	DURATION	CAL. BURNED	CLASS GROUP ACTIVITY
		TOTAL		

TOTAL CALORIES BURNED TODAY _____

COMMENTS ON TODAY'S FOOD AND EXERCISE/GOALS FOR TOMORROW:

_____

_____

_____

_____

_____

_____

_____

CALORIE GOAL _____　　　FAT GOAL _____

FOOD

TIME	AMT.	FOOD	PROTEIN (G)	CARBS (G)	CAL.	CAL. BALANCE	FAT (G)	FAT BALANCE
		TOTALS FOR TODAY						

# of 8-ounce glasses of water drank today:

EXERCISE

STRETCHING / WARMING UP / FLEXIBILITY

TIME	TYPE	DURATION	CAL. BURNED	CLASS GROUP ACTIVITY
		TOTAL		

STRENGTH TRAINING / WEIGHT LIFTING

TIME	TYPE	DURATION	CAL. BURNED	CLASS GROUP ACTIVITY
		TOTAL		

CARDIOVASCULAR

TIME	TYPE	DURATION	CAL. BURNED	CLASS GROUP ACTIVITY
		TOTAL		

TOTAL CALORIES BURNED TODAY _____

COMMENTS ON TODAY'S FOOD AND EXERCISE/GOALS FOR TOMORROW:

_____

_____

_____

_____

_____

_____

_____

_____

DAY 52

CALORIE GOAL _____   **FAT GOAL** _____

FOOD

TIME	AMT.	FOOD	PROTEIN (G)	CARBS (G)	CAL.	CAL. BALANCE	FAT (G)	FAT BALANCE
		TOTALS FOR TODAY						

# of 8-ounce glasses of water drank today:

EXERCISE

STRETCHING / WARMING UP / FLEXIBILITY

TIME	TYPE	DURATION	CAL. BURNED	CLASS GROUP ACTIVITY
		TOTAL		

STRENGTH TRAINING / WEIGHT LIFTING

TIME	TYPE	DURATION	CAL. BURNED	CLASS GROUP ACTIVITY
		TOTAL		

CARDIOVASCULAR

TIME	TYPE	DURATION	CAL. BURNED	CLASS GROUP ACTIVITY
		TOTAL		

TOTAL CALORIES BURNED TODAY _____

COMMENTS ON TODAY'S FOOD AND EXERCISE/GOALS FOR TOMORROW:

_____

_____

_____

_____

_____

_____

_____

_____

DAY 53

CALORIE GOAL _____   FAT GOAL _____

FOOD

TIME	AMT.	FOOD	PROTEIN (G)	CARBS (G)	CAL.	CAL. BALANCE	FAT (G)	FAT BALANCE
		TOTALS FOR TODAY						

# of 8-ounce glasses of water drank today:

EXERCISE

STRETCHING / WARMING UP / FLEXIBILITY

TIME	TYPE	DURATION	CAL. BURNED	CLASS GROUP ACTIVITY
		TOTAL		

STRENGTH TRAINING / WEIGHT LIFTING

TIME	TYPE	DURATION	CAL. BURNED	CLASS GROUP ACTIVITY
		TOTAL		

CARDIOVASCULAR

TIME	TYPE	DURATION	CAL. BURNED	CLASS GROUP ACTIVITY
		TOTAL		

TOTAL CALORIES BURNED TODAY _____

COMMENTS ON TODAY'S FOOD AND EXERCISE/GOALS FOR TOMORROW:

_____

_____

_____

_____

_____

_____

_____

DATE   DAY 54

CALORIE GOAL _____   FAT GOAL _____

FOOD

TIME	AMT.	FOOD	PROTEIN (G)	CARBS (G)	CAL.	CAL. BALANCE	FAT (G)	FAT BALANCE
		TOTALS FOR TODAY						

# of 8-ounce glasses of water drank today:

EXERCISE

STRETCHING / WARMING UP / FLEXIBILITY

TIME	TYPE	DURATION	CAL. BURNED	CLASS GROUP ACTIVITY
	TOTAL			

STRENGTH TRAINING / WEIGHT LIFTING

TIME	TYPE	DURATION	CAL. BURNED	CLASS GROUP ACTIVITY
	TOTAL			

CARDIOVASCULAR

TIME	TYPE	DURATION	CAL. BURNED	CLASS GROUP ACTIVITY
	TOTAL			

TOTAL CALORIES BURNED TODAY _____

COMMENTS ON TODAY'S FOOD AND EXERCISE/GOALS FOR TOMORROW:

_____

_____

_____

_____

_____

_____

_____

_____

DAY 55

CALORIE GOAL _____   FAT GOAL _____

FOOD

TIME	AMT.	FOOD	PROTEIN (G)	CARBS (G)	CAL.	CAL. BALANCE	FAT (G)	FAT BALANCE
		TOTALS FOR TODAY						

# of 8-ounce glasses of water drank today:

EXERCISE

STRETCHING / WARMING UP / FLEXIBILITY

TIME	TYPE	DURATION	CAL. BURNED	CLASS GROUP ACTIVITY
		TOTAL		

STRENGTH TRAINING / WEIGHT LIFTING

TIME	TYPE	DURATION	CAL. BURNED	CLASS GROUP ACTIVITY
		TOTAL		

CARDIOVASCULAR

TIME	TYPE	DURATION	CAL. BURNED	CLASS GROUP ACTIVITY
		TOTAL		

TOTAL CALORIES BURNED TODAY _____

COMMENTS ON TODAY'S FOOD AND EXERCISE/GOALS FOR TOMORROW:

_____

_____

_____

_____

_____

_____

_____

DAY 56

CALORIE GOAL _____ FAT GOAL _____

FOOD

TIME	AMT.	FOOD	PROTEIN (G)	CARBS (G)	CAL.	CAL. BALANCE	FAT (G)	FAT BALANCE
		TOTALS FOR TODAY						

# of 8-ounce glasses of water drank today:

EXERCISE

STRETCHING / WARMING UP / FLEXIBILITY

TIME	TYPE	DURATION	CAL. BURNED	CLASS GROUP ACTIVITY
		TOTAL		

STRENGTH TRAINING / WEIGHT LIFTING

TIME	TYPE	DURATION	CAL. BURNED	CLASS GROUP ACTIVITY
		TOTAL		

CARDIOVASCULAR

TIME	TYPE	DURATION	CAL. BURNED	CLASS GROUP ACTIVITY
		TOTAL		

TOTAL CALORIES BURNED TODAY _____

WEEKLY WEIGH-IN:

ORIGINAL WEIGHT _____ NEW WEIGHT _____ WEIGHT CHANGE _____

POUNDS LEFT BEFORE MY 90-DAY GOAL IS REACHED _____

RECALCULATED DAILY CALORIE BALANCE FOR NEXT WEEK _____

RECALCULATED DAILY FAT BALANCE FOR NEXT WEEK _____

NOTES ABOUT THIS WEEK: _____

_____

_____

_____

CALORIE GOAL _____   **FAT GOAL** _____

FOOD

TIME	AMT.	FOOD	PROTEIN (G)	CARBS (G)	CAL.	CAL. BALANCE	FAT (G)	FAT BALANCE
		TOTALS FOR TODAY						

# of 8-ounce glasses of water drank today:

EXERCISE

STRETCHING / WARMING UP / FLEXIBILITY

TIME	TYPE	DURATION	CAL. BURNED	CLASS GROUP ACTIVITY
	TOTAL			

STRENGTH TRAINING / WEIGHT LIFTING

TIME	TYPE	DURATION	CAL. BURNED	CLASS GROUP ACTIVITY
	TOTAL			

CARDIOVASCULAR

TIME	TYPE	DURATION	CAL. BURNED	CLASS GROUP ACTIVITY
	TOTAL			

TOTAL CALORIES BURNED TODAY _____

COMMENTS ON TODAY'S FOOD AND EXERCISE/GOALS FOR TOMORROW:

_____

_____

_____

_____

_____

_____

_____

DAY 58

CALORIE GOAL _____   FAT GOAL _____

FOOD

TIME	AMT.	FOOD	PROTEIN (G)	CARBS (G)	CAL.	CAL. BALANCE	FAT (G)	FAT BALANCE
		TOTALS FOR TODAY						

# of 8-ounce glasses of water drank today:

EXERCISE

STRETCHING / WARMING UP / FLEXIBILITY

TIME	TYPE	DURATION	CAL. BURNED	CLASS GROUP ACTIVITY
		TOTAL		

STRENGTH TRAINING / WEIGHT LIFTING

TIME	TYPE	DURATION	CAL. BURNED	CLASS GROUP ACTIVITY
		TOTAL		

CARDIOVASCULAR

TIME	TYPE	DURATION	CAL. BURNED	CLASS GROUP ACTIVITY
		TOTAL		

TOTAL CALORIES BURNED TODAY _____

COMMENTS ON TODAY'S FOOD AND EXERCISE/GOALS FOR TOMORROW:

_____

_____

_____

_____

_____

_____

_____

DAY 59

CALORIE GOAL _____ **FAT GOAL** _____

FOOD

TIME	AMT.	FOOD	PROTEIN (G)	CARBS (G)	CAL.	CAL. BALANCE	FAT (G)	FAT BALANCE
		TOTALS FOR TODAY						

# of 8-ounce glasses of water drank today:

EXERCISE

STRETCHING / WARMING UP / FLEXIBILITY

TIME	TYPE	DURATION	CAL. BURNED	CLASS GROUP ACTIVITY
		TOTAL		

STRENGTH TRAINING / WEIGHT LIFTING

TIME	TYPE	DURATION	CAL. BURNED	CLASS GROUP ACTIVITY
		TOTAL		

CARDIOVASCULAR

TIME	TYPE	DURATION	CAL. BURNED	CLASS GROUP ACTIVITY
		TOTAL		

TOTAL CALORIES BURNED TODAY _____

COMMENTS ON TODAY'S FOOD AND EXERCISE/GOALS FOR TOMORROW:

_____

_____

_____

_____

_____

_____

_____

_____

DAY 60

CALORIE GOAL _____   FAT GOAL _____

FOOD

TIME	AMT.	FOOD	PROTEIN (G)	CARBS (G)	CAL.	CAL. BALANCE	FAT (G)	FAT BALANCE
		TOTALS FOR TODAY						

# of 8-ounce glasses of water drank today:

EXERCISE

STRETCHING / WARMING UP / FLEXIBILITY

TIME	TYPE	DURATION	CAL. BURNED	CLASS GROUP ACTIVITY
		TOTAL		

STRENGTH TRAINING / WEIGHT LIFTING

TIME	TYPE	DURATION	CAL. BURNED	CLASS GROUP ACTIVITY
		TOTAL		

CARDIOVASCULAR

TIME	TYPE	DURATION	CAL. BURNED	CLASS GROUP ACTIVITY
		TOTAL		

TOTAL CALORIES BURNED TODAY _____

COMMENTS ON TODAY'S FOOD AND EXERCISE/GOALS FOR TOMORROW:

_____

_____

_____

_____

_____

_____

_____

_____

147

CALORIE GOAL _____ FAT GOAL _____

FOOD

TIME	AMT.	FOOD	PROTEIN (G)	CARBS (G)	CAL.	CAL. BALANCE	FAT (G)	FAT BALANCE
		TOTALS FOR TODAY						

# of 8-ounce glasses of water drank today:

EXERCISE

STRETCHING / WARMING UP / FLEXIBILITY

TIME	TYPE	DURATION	CAL. BURNED	CLASS GROUP ACTIVITY
		TOTAL		

STRENGTH TRAINING / WEIGHT LIFTING

TIME	TYPE	DURATION	CAL. BURNED	CLASS GROUP ACTIVITY
		TOTAL		

CARDIOVASCULAR

TIME	TYPE	DURATION	CAL. BURNED	CLASS GROUP ACTIVITY
		TOTAL		

TOTAL CALORIES BURNED TODAY _____

COMMENTS ON TODAY'S FOOD AND EXERCISE/GOALS FOR TOMORROW:

_____

_____

_____

_____

_____

_____

_____

_____

149

DATE   **DAY 62**

CALORIE GOAL _____   FAT GOAL _____

FOOD

TIME	AMT.	FOOD	PROTEIN (G)	CARBS (G)	CAL.	CAL. BALANCE	FAT (G)	FAT BALANCE
		TOTALS FOR TODAY						

# of 8-ounce glasses of water drank today:

150

EXERCISE

STRETCHING / WARMING UP / FLEXIBILITY

TIME	TYPE	DURATION	CAL. BURNED	CLASS GROUP ACTIVITY
		TOTAL		

STRENGTH TRAINING / WEIGHT LIFTING

TIME	TYPE	DURATION	CAL. BURNED	CLASS GROUP ACTIVITY
		TOTAL		

CARDIOVASCULAR

TIME	TYPE	DURATION	CAL. BURNED	CLASS GROUP ACTIVITY
		TOTAL		

TOTAL CALORIES BURNED TODAY _____

COMMENTS ON TODAY'S FOOD AND EXERCISE/GOALS FOR TOMORROW:

_____

_____

_____

_____

_____

_____

_____

DAY 63

CALORIE GOAL _____   FAT GOAL _____

FOOD

TIME	AMT.	FOOD	PROTEIN (G)	CARBS (G)	CAL.	CAL. BALANCE	FAT (G)	FAT BALANCE
		TOTALS FOR TODAY						

# of 8-ounce glasses of water drank today:

EXERCISE

STRETCHING / WARMING UP / FLEXIBILITY

TIME	TYPE	DURATION	CAL. BURNED	CLASS GROUP ACTIVITY
		TOTAL		

STRENGTH TRAINING / WEIGHT LIFTING

TIME	TYPE	DURATION	CAL. BURNED	CLASS GROUP ACTIVITY
		TOTAL		

CARDIOVASCULAR

TIME	TYPE	DURATION	CAL. BURNED	CLASS GROUP ACTIVITY
		TOTAL		

TOTAL CALORIES BURNED TODAY _____

WEEKLY WEIGH-IN:

ORIGINAL WEIGHT _____ NEW WEIGHT _____ WEIGHT CHANGE _____

POUNDS LEFT BEFORE MY 90-DAY GOAL IS REACHED _____

RECALCULATED DAILY CALORIE BALANCE FOR NEXT WEEK _____

RECALCULATED DAILY FAT BALANCE FOR NEXT WEEK _____

NOTES ABOUT THIS WEEK: _____

_____

_____

_____

DAY 64

CALORIE GOAL _____   **FAT GOAL** _____

FOOD

TIME	AMT.	FOOD	PROTEIN (G)	CARBS (G)	CAL.	CAL. BALANCE	FAT (G)	FAT BALANCE
		TOTALS FOR TODAY						

# of 8-ounce glasses of water drank today:

EXERCISE

STRETCHING / WARMING UP / FLEXIBILITY

TIME	TYPE	DURATION	CAL. BURNED	CLASS GROUP ACTIVITY
		TOTAL		

STRENGTH TRAINING / WEIGHT LIFTING

TIME	TYPE	DURATION	CAL. BURNED	CLASS GROUP ACTIVITY
		TOTAL		

CARDIOVASCULAR

TIME	TYPE	DURATION	CAL. BURNED	CLASS GROUP ACTIVITY
		TOTAL		

TOTAL CALORIES BURNED TODAY _____

COMMENTS ON TODAY'S FOOD AND EXERCISE/GOALS FOR TOMORROW:

_____

_____

_____

_____

_____

_____

_____

_____

DATE _____   **DAY 65**

CALORIE GOAL _____   FAT GOAL _____

FOOD

TIME	AMT.	FOOD	PROTEIN (G)	CARBS (G)	CAL.	CAL. BALANCE	FAT (G)	FAT BALANCE
		TOTALS FOR TODAY						

# of 8-ounce glasses of water drank today:

EXERCISE

STRETCHING / WARMING UP / FLEXIBILITY

TIME	TYPE	DURATION	CAL. BURNED	CLASS GROUP ACTIVITY
		TOTAL		

STRENGTH TRAINING / WEIGHT LIFTING

TIME	TYPE	DURATION	CAL. BURNED	CLASS GROUP ACTIVITY
		TOTAL		

CARDIOVASCULAR

TIME	TYPE	DURATION	CAL. BURNED	CLASS GROUP ACTIVITY
		TOTAL		

TOTAL CALORIES BURNED TODAY _____

COMMENTS ON TODAY'S FOOD AND EXERCISE/GOALS FOR TOMORROW:

_____

_____

_____

_____

_____

_____

_____

DATE

DAY 66

CALORIE GOAL _____   FAT GOAL _____

FOOD

TIME	AMT.	FOOD	PROTEIN (G)	CARBS (G)	CAL.	CAL. BALANCE	FAT (G)	FAT BALANCE
		TOTALS FOR TODAY						

# of 8-ounce glasses of water drank today:

EXERCISE

STRETCHING / WARMING UP / FLEXIBILITY

TIME	TYPE	DURATION	CAL. BURNED	CLASS GROUP ACTIVITY
		TOTAL		

STRENGTH TRAINING / WEIGHT LIFTING

TIME	TYPE	DURATION	CAL. BURNED	CLASS GROUP ACTIVITY
		TOTAL		

CARDIOVASCULAR

TIME	TYPE	DURATION	CAL. BURNED	CLASS GROUP ACTIVITY
		TOTAL		

TOTAL CALORIES BURNED TODAY _____

COMMENTS ON TODAY'S FOOD AND EXERCISE/GOALS FOR TOMORROW:

DATE   DAY 67

CALORIE GOAL _____   FAT GOAL _____

FOOD

TIME	AMT.	FOOD	PROTEIN (G)	CARBS (G)	CAL.	CAL. BALANCE	FAT (G)	FAT BALANCE
		TOTALS FOR TODAY						

# of 8-ounce glasses of water drank today:

EXERCISE

STRETCHING / WARMING UP / FLEXIBILITY

TIME	TYPE	DURATION	CAL. BURNED	CLASS GROUP ACTIVITY
	TOTAL			

STRENGTH TRAINING / WEIGHT LIFTING

TIME	TYPE	DURATION	CAL. BURNED	CLASS GROUP ACTIVITY
	TOTAL			

CARDIOVASCULAR

TIME	TYPE	DURATION	CAL. BURNED	CLASS GROUP ACTIVITY
	TOTAL			

TOTAL CALORIES BURNED TODAY _____

COMMENTS ON TODAY'S FOOD AND EXERCISE/GOALS FOR TOMORROW:

_____

_____

_____

_____

_____

_____

_____

DATE   DAY 68

CALORIE GOAL _____   **FAT GOAL** _____

FOOD

TIME	AMT.	FOOD	PROTEIN (G)	CARBS (G)	CAL.	CAL. BALANCE	FAT (G)	FAT BALANCE
		TOTALS FOR TODAY						

# of 8-ounce glasses of water drank today:

EXERCISE

STRETCHING / WARMING UP / FLEXIBILITY

TIME	TYPE	DURATION	CAL. BURNED	CLASS GROUP ACTIVITY
		TOTAL		

STRENGTH TRAINING / WEIGHT LIFTING

TIME	TYPE	DURATION	CAL. BURNED	CLASS GROUP ACTIVITY
		TOTAL		

CARDIOVASCULAR

TIME	TYPE	DURATION	CAL. BURNED	CLASS GROUP ACTIVITY
		TOTAL		

TOTAL CALORIES BURNED TODAY _____

COMMENTS ON TODAY'S FOOD AND EXERCISE/GOALS FOR TOMORROW:

_____

_____

_____

_____

_____

_____

_____

_____

DAY 69

CALORIE GOAL _____   **FAT GOAL** _____

FOOD

TIME	AMT.	FOOD	PROTEIN (G)	CARBS (G)	CAL.	CAL. BALANCE	FAT (G)	FAT BALANCE
		TOTALS FOR TODAY						

# of 8-ounce glasses of water drank today:

EXERCISE

STRETCHING / WARMING UP / FLEXIBILITY

TIME	TYPE	DURATION	CAL. BURNED	CLASS GROUP ACTIVITY
		TOTAL		

STRENGTH TRAINING / WEIGHT LIFTING

TIME	TYPE	DURATION	CAL. BURNED	CLASS GROUP ACTIVITY
		TOTAL		

CARDIOVASCULAR

TIME	TYPE	DURATION	CAL. BURNED	CLASS GROUP ACTIVITY
		TOTAL		

TOTAL CALORIES BURNED TODAY _____

COMMENTS ON TODAY'S FOOD AND EXERCISE/GOALS FOR TOMORROW:

_____

_____

_____

_____

_____

_____

_____

CALORIE GOAL _____   FAT GOAL _____

FOOD

TIME	AMT.	FOOD	PROTEIN (G)	CARBS (G)	CAL.	CAL. BALANCE	FAT (G)	FAT BALANCE
		TOTALS FOR TODAY						

# of 8-ounce glasses of water drank today:

EXERCISE

STRETCHING / WARMING UP / FLEXIBILITY

TIME	TYPE	DURATION	CAL. BURNED	CLASS GROUP ACTIVITY
		TOTAL		

STRENGTH TRAINING / WEIGHT LIFTING

TIME	TYPE	DURATION	CAL. BURNED	CLASS GROUP ACTIVITY
		TOTAL		

CARDIOVASCULAR

TIME	TYPE	DURATION	CAL. BURNED	CLASS GROUP ACTIVITY
		TOTAL		

TOTAL CALORIES BURNED TODAY _____

WEEKLY WEIGH-IN:

ORIGINAL WEIGHT _____   NEW WEIGHT _____   WEIGHT CHANGE _____

POUNDS LEFT BEFORE MY 90-DAY GOAL IS REACHED _____

RECALCULATED DAILY CALORIE BALANCE FOR NEXT WEEK _____

RECALCULATED DAILY FAT BALANCE FOR NEXT WEEK _____

NOTES ABOUT THIS WEEK: _____

_____

_____

_____

DAY 71

CALORIE GOAL _____   FAT GOAL _____

FOOD

TIME	AMT.	FOOD	PROTEIN (G)	CARBS (G)	CAL.	CAL. BALANCE	FAT (G)	FAT BALANCE
		TOTALS FOR TODAY						

\# of 8-ounce glasses of water drank today:

EXERCISE

STRETCHING / WARMING UP / FLEXIBILITY

TIME	TYPE	DURATION	CAL. BURNED	CLASS GROUP ACTIVITY
		TOTAL		

STRENGTH TRAINING / WEIGHT LIFTING

TIME	TYPE	DURATION	CAL. BURNED	CLASS GROUP ACTIVITY
		TOTAL		

CARDIOVASCULAR

TIME	TYPE	DURATION	CAL. BURNED	CLASS GROUP ACTIVITY
		TOTAL		

TOTAL CALORIES BURNED TODAY _____

COMMENTS ON TODAY'S FOOD AND EXERCISE/GOALS FOR TOMORROW:

_____

_____

_____

_____

_____

_____

_____

CALORIE GOAL _____   FAT GOAL _____

FOOD

TIME	AMT.	FOOD	PROTEIN (G)	CARBS (G)	CAL.	CAL. BALANCE	FAT (G)	FAT BALANCE
		TOTALS FOR TODAY						

# of 8-ounce glasses of water drank today:

EXERCISE

STRETCHING / WARMING UP / FLEXIBILITY

TIME	TYPE	DURATION	CAL. BURNED	CLASS GROUP ACTIVITY
		TOTAL		

STRENGTH TRAINING / WEIGHT LIFTING

TIME	TYPE	DURATION	CAL. BURNED	CLASS GROUP ACTIVITY
		TOTAL		

CARDIOVASCULAR

TIME	TYPE	DURATION	CAL. BURNED	CLASS GROUP ACTIVITY
		TOTAL		

TOTAL CALORIES BURNED TODAY _____

COMMENTS ON TODAY'S FOOD AND EXERCISE/GOALS FOR TOMORROW:

_____

_____

_____

_____

_____

_____

_____

DATE   DAY 73

CALORIE GOAL _____   FAT GOAL _____

FOOD

TIME	AMT.	FOOD	PROTEIN (G)	CARBS (G)	CAL.	CAL. BALANCE	FAT (G)	FAT BALANCE
		TOTALS FOR TODAY						

# of 8-ounce glasses of water drank today:

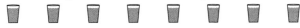

172

EXERCISE

STRETCHING / WARMING UP / FLEXIBILITY

TIME	TYPE	DURATION	CAL. BURNED	CLASS GROUP ACTIVITY
		TOTAL		

STRENGTH TRAINING / WEIGHT LIFTING

TIME	TYPE	DURATION	CAL. BURNED	CLASS GROUP ACTIVITY
		TOTAL		

CARDIOVASCULAR

TIME	TYPE	DURATION	CAL. BURNED	CLASS GROUP ACTIVITY
		TOTAL		

TOTAL CALORIES BURNED TODAY _____

COMMENTS ON TODAY'S FOOD AND EXERCISE/GOALS FOR TOMORROW:

_____

_____

_____

_____

_____

_____

_____

DATE   **DAY 74**

CALORIE GOAL _____   FAT GOAL _____

FOOD

TIME	AMT.	FOOD	PROTEIN (G)	CARBS (G)	CAL.	CAL. BALANCE	FAT (G)	FAT BALANCE
		TOTALS FOR TODAY						

# of 8-ounce glasses of water drank today:

174

EXERCISE

STRETCHING / WARMING UP / FLEXIBILITY

TIME	TYPE	DURATION	CAL. BURNED	CLASS GROUP ACTIVITY
		TOTAL		

STRENGTH TRAINING / WEIGHT LIFTING

TIME	TYPE	DURATION	CAL. BURNED	CLASS GROUP ACTIVITY
		TOTAL		

CARDIOVASCULAR

TIME	TYPE	DURATION	CAL. BURNED	CLASS GROUP ACTIVITY
		TOTAL		

TOTAL CALORIES BURNED TODAY _____

COMMENTS ON TODAY'S FOOD AND EXERCISE/GOALS FOR TOMORROW:

_____

_____

_____

_____

_____

_____

_____

_____

CALORIE GOAL _____   **FAT GOAL** _____

FOOD

TIME	AMT.	FOOD	PROTEIN (G)	CARBS (G)	CAL.	CAL. BALANCE	FAT (G)	FAT BALANCE
		TOTALS FOR TODAY						

# of 8-ounce glasses of water drank today:

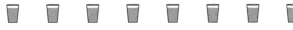

EXERCISE

STRETCHING / WARMING UP / FLEXIBILITY

TIME	TYPE	DURATION	CAL. BURNED	CLASS GROUP ACTIVITY
		TOTAL		

STRENGTH TRAINING / WEIGHT LIFTING

TIME	TYPE	DURATION	CAL. BURNED	CLASS GROUP ACTIVITY
		TOTAL		

CARDIOVASCULAR

TIME	TYPE	DURATION	CAL. BURNED	CLASS GROUP ACTIVITY
		TOTAL		

TOTAL CALORIES BURNED TODAY _____

COMMENTS ON TODAY'S FOOD AND EXERCISE/GOALS FOR TOMORROW:

_____

_____

_____

_____

_____

_____

_____

_____

DAY 76

CALORIE GOAL _____   FAT GOAL _____

FOOD

TIME	AMT.	FOOD	PROTEIN (G)	CARBS (G)	CAL.	CAL. BALANCE	FAT (G)	FAT BALANCE
		TOTALS FOR TODAY						

# of 8-ounce glasses of water drank today:

EXERCISE

STRETCHING / WARMING UP / FLEXIBILITY

TIME	TYPE	DURATION	CAL. BURNED	CLASS GROUP ACTIVITY
		TOTAL		

STRENGTH TRAINING / WEIGHT LIFTING

TIME	TYPE	DURATION	CAL. BURNED	CLASS GROUP ACTIVITY
		TOTAL		

CARDIOVASCULAR

TIME	TYPE	DURATION	CAL. BURNED	CLASS GROUP ACTIVITY
		TOTAL		

TOTAL CALORIES BURNED TODAY _____

COMMENTS ON TODAY'S FOOD AND EXERCISE/GOALS FOR TOMORROW:

_____

_____

_____

_____

_____

_____

_____

_____

CALORIE GOAL _____   FAT GOAL _____

FOOD

TIME	AMT.	FOOD	PROTEIN (G)	CARBS (G)	CAL.	CAL. BALANCE	FAT (G)	FAT BALANCE
		TOTALS FOR TODAY						

# of 8-ounce glasses of water drank today:

EXERCISE

STRETCHING / WARMING UP / FLEXIBILITY

TIME	TYPE	DURATION	CAL. BURNED	CLASS GROUP ACTIVITY
		TOTAL		

STRENGTH TRAINING / WEIGHT LIFTING

TIME	TYPE	DURATION	CAL. BURNED	CLASS GROUP ACTIVITY
		TOTAL		

CARDIOVASCULAR

TIME	TYPE	DURATION	CAL. BURNED	CLASS GROUP ACTIVITY
		TOTAL		

TOTAL CALORIES BURNED TODAY _____

WEEKLY WEIGH-IN:

ORIGINAL WEIGHT _____   NEW WEIGHT _____   WEIGHT CHANGE _____

POUNDS LEFT BEFORE MY 90-DAY GOAL IS REACHED _____

RECALCULATED DAILY CALORIE BALANCE FOR NEXT WEEK _____

RECALCULATED DAILY FAT BALANCE FOR NEXT WEEK _____

NOTES ABOUT THIS WEEK: _____

_____

_____

_____

CALORIE GOAL _____   FAT GOAL _____

FOOD

TIME	AMT.	FOOD	PROTEIN (G)	CARBS (G)	CAL.	CAL. BALANCE	FAT (G)	FAT BALANCE
		TOTALS FOR TODAY						

# of 8-ounce glasses of water drank today:

EXERCISE

STRETCHING / WARMING UP / FLEXIBILITY

TIME	TYPE	DURATION	CAL. BURNED	CLASS GROUP ACTIVITY
		TOTAL		

STRENGTH TRAINING / WEIGHT LIFTING

TIME	TYPE	DURATION	CAL. BURNED	CLASS GROUP ACTIVITY
		TOTAL		

CARDIOVASCULAR

TIME	TYPE	DURATION	CAL. BURNED	CLASS GROUP ACTIVITY
		TOTAL		

TOTAL CALORIES BURNED TODAY _____

COMMENTS ON TODAY'S FOOD AND EXERCISE/GOALS FOR TOMORROW:

_____

_____

_____

_____

_____

_____

_____

_____

CALORIE GOAL _____   FAT GOAL _____

FOOD

TIME	AMT.	FOOD	PROTEIN (G)	CARBS (G)	CAL.	CAL. BALANCE	FAT (G)	FAT BALANCE
		TOTALS FOR TODAY						

# of 8-ounce glasses of water drank today:

EXERCISE

STRETCHING / WARMING UP / FLEXIBILITY

TIME	TYPE	DURATION	CAL. BURNED	CLASS GROUP ACTIVITY
		TOTAL		

STRENGTH TRAINING / WEIGHT LIFTING

TIME	TYPE	DURATION	CAL. BURNED	CLASS GROUP ACTIVITY
		TOTAL		

CARDIOVASCULAR

TIME	TYPE	DURATION	CAL. BURNED	CLASS GROUP ACTIVITY
		TOTAL		

TOTAL CALORIES BURNED TODAY _____

COMMENTS ON TODAY'S FOOD AND EXERCISE/GOALS FOR TOMORROW:

_____

_____

_____

_____

_____

_____

_____

_____

CALORIE GOAL _____   **FAT GOAL** _____

FOOD

TIME	AMT.	FOOD	PROTEIN (G)	CARBS (G)	CAL.	CAL. BALANCE	FAT (G)	FAT BALANCE
		TOTALS FOR TODAY						

# of 8-ounce glasses of water drank today:

EXERCISE

STRETCHING / WARMING UP / FLEXIBILITY

TIME	TYPE	DURATION	CAL. BURNED	CLASS GROUP ACTIVITY
		TOTAL		

STRENGTH TRAINING / WEIGHT LIFTING

TIME	TYPE	DURATION	CAL. BURNED	CLASS GROUP ACTIVITY
		TOTAL		

CARDIOVASCULAR

TIME	TYPE	DURATION	CAL. BURNED	CLASS GROUP ACTIVITY
		TOTAL		

TOTAL CALORIES BURNED TODAY _____

COMMENTS ON TODAY'S FOOD AND EXERCISE/GOALS FOR TOMORROW:

_____

_____

_____

_____

_____

_____

_____

_____

DAY 81

CALORIE GOAL _____ **FAT GOAL** _____

FOOD

TIME	AMT.	FOOD	PROTEIN (G)	CARBS (G)	CAL.	CAL. BALANCE	FAT (G)	FAT BALANCE
		TOTALS FOR TODAY						

# of 8-ounce glasses of water drank today:

EXERCISE

STRETCHING / WARMING UP / FLEXIBILITY

TIME	TYPE	DURATION	CAL. BURNED	CLASS GROUP ACTIVITY
		TOTAL		

STRENGTH TRAINING / WEIGHT LIFTING

TIME	TYPE	DURATION	CAL. BURNED	CLASS GROUP ACTIVITY
		TOTAL		

CARDIOVASCULAR

TIME	TYPE	DURATION	CAL. BURNED	CLASS GROUP ACTIVITY
		TOTAL		

TOTAL CALORIES BURNED TODAY _____

COMMENTS ON TODAY'S FOOD AND EXERCISE/GOALS FOR TOMORROW:

_____

_____

_____

_____

_____

_____

_____

_____

DAY 82

CALORIE GOAL _____   FAT GOAL _____

FOOD

TIME	AMT.	FOOD	PROTEIN (G)	CARBS (G)	CAL.	CAL. BALANCE	FAT (G)	FAT BALANCE
	TOTALS FOR TODAY							

# of 8-ounce glasses of water drank today:

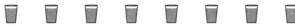

EXERCISE

STRETCHING / WARMING UP / FLEXIBILITY

TIME	TYPE	DURATION	CAL. BURNED	CLASS GROUP ACTIVITY
		TOTAL		

STRENGTH TRAINING / WEIGHT LIFTING

TIME	TYPE	DURATION	CAL. BURNED	CLASS GROUP ACTIVITY
		TOTAL		

CARDIOVASCULAR

TIME	TYPE	DURATION	CAL. BURNED	CLASS GROUP ACTIVITY
		TOTAL		

TOTAL CALORIES BURNED TODAY _____

COMMENTS ON TODAY'S FOOD AND EXERCISE/GOALS FOR TOMORROW:

_____

_____

_____

_____

_____

_____

_____

DAY 83

CALORIE GOAL _____ **FAT GOAL** _____

FOOD

TIME	AMT.	FOOD	PROTEIN (G)	CARBS (G)	CAL.	CAL. BALANCE	FAT (G)	FAT BALANCE
		TOTALS FOR TODAY						

# of 8-ounce glasses of water drank today:

EXERCISE

STRETCHING / WARMING UP / FLEXIBILITY

TIME	TYPE	DURATION	CAL. BURNED	CLASS GROUP ACTIVITY
		TOTAL		

STRENGTH TRAINING / WEIGHT LIFTING

TIME	TYPE	DURATION	CAL. BURNED	CLASS GROUP ACTIVITY
		TOTAL		

CARDIOVASCULAR

TIME	TYPE	DURATION	CAL. BURNED	CLASS GROUP ACTIVITY
		TOTAL		

TOTAL CALORIES BURNED TODAY _____

COMMENTS ON TODAY'S FOOD AND EXERCISE/GOALS FOR TOMORROW:

_____

_____

_____

_____

_____

_____

_____

DAY 84

CALORIE GOAL _____ **FAT GOAL** _____

FOOD

TIME	AMT.	FOOD	PROTEIN (G)	CARBS (G)	CAL.	CAL. BALANCE	FAT (G)	FAT BALANCE
		TOTALS FOR TODAY						

# of 8-ounce glasses of water drank today:

EXERCISE

STRETCHING / WARMING UP / FLEXIBILITY

TIME	TYPE	DURATION	CAL. BURNED	CLASS GROUP ACTIVITY
		TOTAL		

STRENGTH TRAINING / WEIGHT LIFTING

TIME	TYPE	DURATION	CAL. BURNED	CLASS GROUP ACTIVITY
		TOTAL		

CARDIOVASCULAR

TIME	TYPE	DURATION	CAL. BURNED	CLASS GROUP ACTIVITY
		TOTAL		

TOTAL CALORIES BURNED TODAY _____

WEEKLY WEIGH-IN:

ORIGINAL WEIGHT _____   NEW WEIGHT _____   WEIGHT CHANGE _____

POUNDS LEFT BEFORE MY 90-DAY GOAL IS REACHED _____

RECALCULATED DAILY CALORIE BALANCE FOR NEXT WEEK _____

RECALCULATED DAILY FAT BALANCE FOR NEXT WEEK _____

NOTES ABOUT THIS WEEK: _____

_____

_____

_____

DAY 85

CALORIE GOAL _____   FAT GOAL _____

FOOD

TIME	AMT.	FOOD	PROTEIN (G)	CARBS (G)	CAL.	CAL. BALANCE	FAT (G)	FAT BALANCE
		TOTALS FOR TODAY						

# of 8-ounce glasses of water drank today:

EXERCISE

STRETCHING / WARMING UP / FLEXIBILITY

TIME	TYPE	DURATION	CAL. BURNED	CLASS GROUP ACTIVITY
		TOTAL		

STRENGTH TRAINING / WEIGHT LIFTING

TIME	TYPE	DURATION	CAL. BURNED	CLASS GROUP ACTIVITY
		TOTAL		

CARDIOVASCULAR

TIME	TYPE	DURATION	CAL. BURNED	CLASS GROUP ACTIVITY
		TOTAL		

TOTAL CALORIES BURNED TODAY _____

COMMENTS ON TODAY'S FOOD AND EXERCISE/GOALS FOR TOMORROW:

_____

_____

_____

_____

_____

_____

_____

_____

DAY 86

CALORIE GOAL _____   **FAT GOAL** _____

FOOD

TIME	AMT.	FOOD	PROTEIN (G)	CARBS (G)	CAL.	CAL. BALANCE	FAT (G)	FAT BALANCE
		TOTALS FOR TODAY						

# of 8-ounce glasses of water drank today:

EXERCISE

STRETCHING / WARMING UP / FLEXIBILITY

TIME	TYPE	DURATION	CAL. BURNED	CLASS GROUP ACTIVITY
		TOTAL		

STRENGTH TRAINING / WEIGHT LIFTING

TIME	TYPE	DURATION	CAL. BURNED	CLASS GROUP ACTIVITY
		TOTAL		

CARDIOVASCULAR

TIME	TYPE	DURATION	CAL. BURNED	CLASS GROUP ACTIVITY
		TOTAL		

TOTAL CALORIES BURNED TODAY _____

COMMENTS ON TODAY'S FOOD AND EXERCISE/GOALS FOR TOMORROW:

_____

_____

_____

_____

_____

_____

_____

_____

DATE

DAY 87

CALORIE GOAL _____   FAT GOAL _____

FOOD

TIME	AMT.	FOOD	PROTEIN (G)	CARBS (G)	CAL.	CAL. BALANCE	FAT (G)	FAT BALANCE
		TOTALS FOR TODAY						

# of 8-ounce glasses of water drank today:

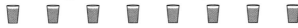

EXERCISE

STRETCHING / WARMING UP / FLEXIBILITY

TIME	TYPE	DURATION	CAL. BURNED	CLASS GROUP ACTIVITY
		TOTAL		

STRENGTH TRAINING / WEIGHT LIFTING

TIME	TYPE	DURATION	CAL. BURNED	CLASS GROUP ACTIVITY
		TOTAL		

CARDIOVASCULAR

TIME	TYPE	DURATION	CAL. BURNED	CLASS GROUP ACTIVITY
		TOTAL		

TOTAL CALORIES BURNED TODAY _____

COMMENTS ON TODAY'S FOOD AND EXERCISE/GOALS FOR TOMORROW:

_____

_____

_____

_____

_____

_____

_____

CALORIE GOAL _____   FAT GOAL _____

FOOD

TIME	AMT.	FOOD	PROTEIN (G)	CARBS (G)	CAL.	CAL. BALANCE	FAT (G)	FAT BALANCE
		TOTALS FOR TODAY						

# of 8-ounce glasses of water drank today:

EXERCISE

STRETCHING / WARMING UP / FLEXIBILITY

TIME	TYPE	DURATION	CAL. BURNED	CLASS GROUP ACTIVITY
	TOTAL			

STRENGTH TRAINING / WEIGHT LIFTING

TIME	TYPE	DURATION	CAL. BURNED	CLASS GROUP ACTIVITY
	TOTAL			

CARDIOVASCULAR

TIME	TYPE	DURATION	CAL. BURNED	CLASS GROUP ACTIVITY
	TOTAL			

TOTAL CALORIES BURNED TODAY _____

COMMENTS ON TODAY'S FOOD AND EXERCISE/GOALS FOR TOMORROW:

_____

_____

_____

_____

_____

_____

_____

_____

DATE   **DAY 89**

CALORIE GOAL _____   FAT GOAL _____

FOOD

TIME	AMT.	FOOD	PROTEIN (G)	CARBS (G)	CAL.	CAL. BALANCE	FAT (G)	FAT BALANCE
		TOTALS FOR TODAY						

# of 8-ounce glasses of water drank today:

EXERCISE

STRETCHING / WARMING UP / FLEXIBILITY

TIME	TYPE	DURATION	CAL. BURNED	CLASS GROUP ACTIVITY
		TOTAL		

STRENGTH TRAINING / WEIGHT LIFTING

TIME	TYPE	DURATION	CAL. BURNED	CLASS GROUP ACTIVITY
		TOTAL		

CARDIOVASCULAR

TIME	TYPE	DURATION	CAL. BURNED	CLASS GROUP ACTIVITY
		TOTAL		

TOTAL CALORIES BURNED TODAY _____

COMMENTS ON TODAY'S FOOD AND EXERCISE/GOALS FOR TOMORROW:

_____

_____

_____

_____

_____

_____

_____

_____

DAY 90

CALORIE GOAL _____   FAT GOAL _____

FOOD

TIME	AMT.	FOOD	PROTEIN (G)	CARBS (G)	CAL.	CAL. BALANCE	FAT (G)	FAT BALANCE
		TOTALS FOR TODAY						

# of 8-ounce glasses of water drank today:

EXERCISE

STRETCHING / WARMING UP / FLEXIBILITY

TIME	TYPE	DURATION	CAL. BURNED	CLASS GROUP ACTIVITY
		TOTAL		

STRENGTH TRAINING / WEIGHT LIFTING

TIME	TYPE	DURATION	CAL. BURNED	CLASS GROUP ACTIVITY
		TOTAL		

CARDIOVASCULAR

TIME	TYPE	DURATION	CAL. BURNED	CLASS GROUP ACTIVITY
		TOTAL		

TOTAL CALORIES BURNED TODAY _____

WEEKLY WEIGH-IN:

ORIGINAL WEIGHT _____ NEW WEIGHT _____ WEIGHT CHANGE _____

POUNDS LEFT BEFORE MY 90-DAY GOAL IS REACHED _____

RECALCULATED DAILY CALORIE BALANCE FOR NEXT WEEK _____

RECALCULATED DAILY FAT BALANCE FOR NEXT WEEK _____

NOTES ABOUT THIS WEEK: _____

_____

_____

_____

FAT AND CALORIE CHART
NUTRITIONAL VALUE OF FOODS[3]

FOOD	AMOUNT	CALORIES	FAT (G)	SATURATED FAT (G)
BEVERAGES				
ALCOHOLIC				
Beer				
Regular	12 fl. oz.	146	0	0
Light	12 fl. oz.	99	0	0
Gin, rum, vodka, whiskey				
80 proof	1.5 fl. oz.	97	0	0
86 proof	1.5 fl. oz.	105	0	0
90 proof	1.5 fl. oz.	110	0	0
Mixed drinks				
Daiquiri	2 fl. oz.	112	trace	trace
Pina colada	4.5 fl. oz.	262	3	1.2
Wine				
Dessert				
Dry	3.5 fl. oz.	130	0	0
Sweet	3.5 fl. oz.	158	0	0
Table				
Red	3.5 fl. oz.	74	0	0
White	3.5 fl. oz.	70	0	0
CARBONATED				
Club soda	12 fl. oz.	0	0	0
Cola type	12 fl. oz.	152	0	0
Diet, sweetened with aspartame				
Cola	12 fl. oz.	4	0	0
Other than cola	12 fl. oz.	0	0	0
Ginger ale	12 fl. oz.	124	0	0
Grape	12 fl. oz.	160	0	0

3. Information in this section is taken from "Nutritive Value of Foods, Home and Garden Bulletin Number 72"
United States Department of Agriculture
Agricultural Research Service

FOOD	AMOUNT	CALORIES	FAT (G)	SATURATED FAT (G)
Lemon lime	12 fl. oz.	147	0	0
Orange	12 fl. oz.	179	0	0
Pepper type	12 fl. oz.	151	0	0.3
Root beer	12 fl. oz.	152	0	0

CHOCOLATE-FLAVORED BEVERAGE MIX

Powder	2-3 tsp.	75	1	0.4
Prepared with milk	1 cup	226	9	5.5

COFFEE

Brewed	6 fl. oz.	4	0	trace
Espresso	2 fl. oz.	5	trace	0.1
Instant, prepared	6 fl. oz.	4	0	trace

FRUIT DRINKS

Cranberry juice	8 fl. oz.	144	trace	trace
Fruit punch drink	8 fl. oz.	117	0	trace
Grape drink	8 fl. oz.	113	0	trace
Pineapple-grapefruit juice drink	8 fl. oz.	118	trace	trace
Pineapple-orange juice drink	8 fl. oz.	125	0	0

MILK AND MILK BEVERAGES: See Dairy Products

SOYMILK: See Legumes, Nuts, and Seeds

TEA

Brewed

Black	6 fl. oz.	2	0	trace
Chamomile	6 fl. oz.	2	0	trace

FAT AND CALORIE CHART

FOOD	AMOUNT	CALORIES	FAT (G)	SATURATED FAT (G)

DAIRY PRODUCTS

BUTTER: SEE FATS AND OILS

CHEESE / NATURAL

FOOD	AMOUNT	CALORIES	FAT (G)	SATURATED FAT (G)
Blue	1 oz.	10	8	5.3
Camembert	1.32 oz.	114	9	5.8
Cheddar				
Cut pieces	1 oz.	114	8	6
Shredded	1 cup	455	37	23.8
Cottage				
Creamed (4% fat)				
Large-curd	1 cup	233	10	6.4
Small-curd	1 cup	217	9	6.0
With fruit	1 cup	279	8	4.9
Low-fat (2%)	1 cup	203	4	2.8
Low-fat (1%)	1 cup	164	2	1.5
Uncreamed (dry curd, less than ½% fat)				
	1 cup	123	1	0.4
Cream				
Regular	1 oz.	99	10	6.2
	1 tbsp.	51	5	3.2
Low-fat	1 tbsp.	35	3	1.7
Fat-free	1 tbsp.	15	trace	0.1
Feta	1 oz.	75	6	4.2
Low-fat, Cheddar or Colby	1 oz.	49	2	1.2
Mozzarella				
Whole milk	1 oz.	80	6	3.7
Part-skim milk (low moisture)	1 oz.	79	5	3.1
Muenster	1 oz.	104	9	5.4
Neufchatel	1 oz.	74	7	4.2

FOOD	AMOUNT	CALORIES	FAT (G)	SATURATED FAT (G)
Parmesan, grated	1 cup	456	30	19.1
	1 tbsp.	23	2	1
	1 oz.	129	9	5.4
Provolone	1 oz.	10	8	4.8
Ricotta, made with				
Whole milk	1 cup	428	32	20.4
Part-skim milk	1 cup	340	19	12.1
Swiss	1 oz.	107	8	5
CREAM, SWEET				
Half and half	1 cup	315	28	17.3
	1 tbsp.	20	2	1.1
Light, coffee, or table	1 cup	469	46	28.8
	1 tbsp.	29	3	1.8
Whipped topping (pressurized)	1 cup	154	13	8.3
	1 tbsp.	8	1	0.4
CREAM, SOUR				
Regular	1 cup	493	48	3
	1 tbsp.	26	3	1.6
Reduced-fat	1 tbsp.	20	2	1.1
Fat-free	1 tbsp.	12	0	0
FROZEN DESSERT				
Frozen yogurt, soft-serve				
Chocolate	½ cup	115	4	2.6
Vanilla	½ cup	114	4	2.5
Ice cream				
Regular				
Chocolate	½ cup	143	7	4.5
Vanilla	½ cup	133	7	4.5

FAT AND CALORIE CHART

FOOD	AMOUNT	CALORIES	FAT (G)	SATURATED FAT (G)
50% reduced-fat vanilla	½ cup	92	3	1.7
Low-fat, chocolate	½ cup	113	2	1
Rich, vanilla	½ cup	178	12	7.4
Soft-serve, vanilla	½ cup	185	11	6.4
Sherbet, orange	½ cup	102	1	0.9
MILK				
Whole (33% fat)	1 cup	150	8	5.1
Reduced-fat (2%)	1 cup	121	5	2.9
Low-fat (1%)	1 cup	102	3	1.6
Non-fat (skim)	1 cup	86	trace	0.3
Buttermilk	1 cup	99	2	1.3
Canned				
Condensed, sweetened	1 cup	982	27	16.8
Evaporated				
Whole milk	1 cup	339	19	11.6
Skim milk	1 cup	199	1	0.3
Dried				
Buttermilk	1 cup	464	7	4.3
Non-fat, instant	1 cup	244	trace	0.3
EGG				
RAW				
Whole	1 medium	66	4	1.4
	1 large	75	5	1.6
	1 extra large	86	6	1.8
White	1 large	17	0	0
Yolk	1 large	59	5	1.6
Cooked, whole				
Fried, in margarine, with salt	1 large	92	7	1.9
Hard cooked, shell removed	1 large	78	6	1.6

FOOD	AMOUNT	CALORIES	FAT (G)	SATURATED FAT (G)
Poached, with salt	1 large	75	5	1.5
Scrambled, in margarine, with whole milk, salt				
	1 large	101	7	2.2
Egg substitute	¼ cup	53	2	0.4

FATS AND OILS
BUTTER (4 STICKS/LB.)

FOOD	AMOUNT	CALORIES	FAT (G)	SATURATED FAT (G)
Salted	1 stick	813	92	57.3
	1 tbsp.	102	12	7.2
	1 tsp.	36	4	2.5
Unsalted	1 stick	813	92	57.3
Lard	1 cup	1,849	205	80.4
	1 tbsp.	115	13	5

MARGARINE
Regular (about 80% fat)

FOOD	AMOUNT	CALORIES	FAT (G)	SATURATED FAT (G)
Hard (4 sticks/lb.)	1 stick	815	91	17.9
	1 tbsp.	101	11	2.2
	1 tsp.	34	4	0.7
Soft	1 cup	1,626	183	31.3
	1 tsp.	34	4	0.6
Spread (about 40% fat)	1 cup	801	90	17.9
	1 tsp.	17	2	0.4
Margarine-butter blend	1 stick	811	91	32.1
	1 tbsp.	102	11	4

OILS, SALAD OR COOKING

FOOD	AMOUNT	CALORIES	FAT (G)	SATURATED FAT (G)
Canola	1 tbsp.	124	14	1
Corn	1 tbsp.	120	14	1.7
Olive	1 tbsp.	119	14	1.8
Peanut	1 tbsp.	119	14	2.3

FAT AND CALORIE CHART

FOOD	AMOUNT	CALORIES	FAT (G)	SATURATED FAT (G)
Safflower, high-oleic	1 tbsp.	120	14	0.8
Sesame	1 tbsp.	120	14	1.9
Soybean, hydrogenated	1 tbsp.	120	14	2
Soybean, hydrogenated and cottonseed oil blend				
	1 tbsp.	120	14	2.4
Sunflower	1 tbsp.	120	14	1.4

SALAD DRESSINGS / COMMERCIAL

Blue cheese

Regular	1 tbsp.	77	8	1.5
Low-calorie	1 tbsp.	15	1	0.4

Caesar

Regular	1 tbsp.	78	8	1.3
Low-calorie	1 tbsp.	17	1	0.1

French

Regular	1 tbsp.	67	6	1.5
Low-calorie	1 tbsp.	22	1	0.1

Italian

Regular	1 tbsp.	69	7	1.0
Low-calorie	1 tbsp.	16	1	0.2

Mayonnaise

Regular	1 tbsp.	99	11	1.6
Fat-free	1 tbsp.	12	trace	0.1

Russian

Regular	1 tbsp.	76	8	1.1
Low-calorie	1 tbsp.	23	1	0.1

Thousand Island

Regular	1 tbsp.	59	6	0.9
Low-calorie	1 tbsp.	24	2	0.2
Vinegar and oil	1 tbsp.	70	8	1.4

FOOD	AMOUNT	CALORIES	FAT (G)	SATURATED FAT (G)
FISH AND SHELLFISH				
Catfish, breaded, fried	3 oz.	195	11	2.8
Clam				
Raw, meat only	3 oz.	63	1	0.1
	1 medium	11	trace	trace
Breaded, fried	¾ cup	451	26	6.6
Canned, drained solids	3 oz.	126	2	0.2
	1 cup	237	3	0.3
Cod				
Baked or broiled	3 oz.	89	1	0.1
Canned, solids and liquid	3 oz.	89	1	0.1
Crab				
Alaska King				
Steamed	1 leg	130	2	0.2
	3 oz.	82	1	0.1
Imitation	3 oz.	87	1	0.2
Blue				
Steamed	3 oz.	87	2	0.2
Canned	1 cup	134	2	0.3
Crab cake, with egg, onion, fried in margarine				
	1 cake	93	5	0.9
Fish fillet, battered or breaded, fried				
	1 fillet	211	11	2.6
Fish stick and portion, breaded	1 stick	76	3	0.9
Flounder or sole, baked or broiled	3 oz.	99	1	0.3
	1 fillet	149	2	0.5
Haddock, baked or broiled	3 oz.	95	1	0.1
	1 fillet	168	1	0.3
Halibut, baked or broiled	3 oz.	119	2	0.4
	½ fillet	223	5	0.7
Herring, pickled	3 oz.	223	15	2

FAT AND CALORIE CHART

FOOD	AMOUNT	CALORIES	FAT (G)	SATURATED FAT (G)
Lobster, steamed	3 oz.	83	1	0.1
Ocean perch, baked or broiled	3 oz.	103	2	0.3
	1 fillet	61	1	0.2
Oyster				
Raw, meat only	1 cup	169	6	1.9
	6 medium	57	2	0.6
Breaded, fried	3 oz.	167	11	2.7
Pollock, baked or broiled	3 oz.	96	1	0.2
	1 fillet	68	1	0.1
Rockfish, baked or broiled	3 oz.	103	2	0.4
	1 fillet	180	3	0.7
Roughy, orange, baked or broiled	3 oz.	76	1	trace
Salmon				
Baked or broiled	3 oz.	184	9	1.6
	½ fillet	335	17	3.0
Canned (pink)	3 oz.	118	5	1.3
Smoked (Chinook)	3 oz.	99	4	0.8
Sardine, Atlantic, canned in oil, drained solids				
	3 oz.	177	10	1.3
Scallop				
Breaded, fried	6 large	20	10	2.5
Steamed	3 oz.	95	1	0.1
Shrimp				
Breaded, fried	3 oz.	206	10	1.8
	6 large	109	6	0.9
Canned	3 oz.	102	2	0.3
Swordfish, baked or broiled	3 oz.	132	4	1.2
	1 piece	164	5	1.5
Trout, baked or broiled	3 oz.	144	6	1.8
	1 fillet	120	5	1.5

FOOD	AMOUNT	CALORIES	FAT (G)	SATURATED FAT (G)
Tuna				
Baked or broiled	3 oz.	118	1	0.3
Canned				
Oil-pack, light	3 oz.	168	7	1.3
Water-pack, light	3 oz.	99	1	0.2
Water-pack, solid	3 oz.	109	3	0.7
FRUITS AND FRUIT JUICES				
Apples				
Raw				
Unpeeled	1 apple	81	trace	0.1
Peeled, sliced	1 cup	63	trace	0.1
Dried	5 rings	78	trace	trace
Apple juice	1 cup	117	trace	trace
Applesauce, canned				
Sweetened	1 cup	194	trace	0.1
Unsweetened	1 cup	105	trace	trace
Apricots				
Raw	1 apricot	17	trace	trace
Canned				
Heavy syrup pack	1 cup	214	trace	trace
Dried, sulfured	10 halves	83	trace	trace
Asian pear, raw				
2¼" high x 2½"	1 pear	51	trace	trace
3³⁄₈" high x 3"	1 pear	116	1	trace
Avocados, raw, without skin and seed				
California (about ⅕ whole)	1 oz.	50	5	0.7
Florida (about ¹⁄₁₀ whole)	1 oz.	32	3	0.5
Bananas, raw				
Whole, medium	1 banana	109	1	0.2
Blackberries, raw	1 cup	75	1	trace

FAT AND CALORIE CHART

FOOD	AMOUNT	CALORIES	FAT (G)	SATURATED FAT (G)
Blueberries				
Raw	1 cup	81	1	trace
Frozen, sweetened, thawed	1 cup	186	trace	trace
Cantaloupe (5" diameter)				
Wedge	⅛ melon	24	trace	trace
Cubes	1 cup	56	trace	0.1
Carambola (starfruit), raw				
Whole (3⅝" long)	1 fruit	30	trace	trace
Sliced	1 cup	36	trace	trace
Cherries				
Sour, red, pitted, canned, water-pack				
	1 cup	88	trace	0.1
Sweet, raw, without pits and stems				
	10 cherries	49	1	0.1
Cranberries				
Dried, sweetened	¼ cup	92	trace	trace
Cranberry sauce, sweetened, canned (about 8 slices per can)				
	1 slice	86	trace	trace
Dates, without pits				
Whole	5 dates	116	trace	0.1
Chopped	1 cup	490	1	0.3
Figs, dried	2 figs	97	trace	0.1
Fruit cocktail, canned, fruit and liquid				
Heavy syrup pack	1 cup	181	trace	trace
Juice pack	1 cup	109	trace	trace
Grapefruit				
Pink or red	½ grapefruit	37	trace	trace
Canned, sections with light syrup				
	1 cup	152	trace	trace

FOOD	AMOUNT	CALORIES	FAT (G)	SATURATED FAT (G)
Grapefruit juice				
Raw				
Pink	1 cup	96	trace	trace
White	1 cup	96	trace	trace
Canned				
Unsweetened	1 cup	94	trace	trace
Sweetened	1 cup	115	trace	trace
Grapes, raw	10 grapes	36	trace	0.1
	1 cup	114	1	0.3
Honeydew (6"-7" diameter)				
Wedge	1/8 melon	56	trace	trace
Diced	1 cup	60	trace	trace
Kiwi fruit raw without skin	1 medium	46	trace	trace
Lemons				
Raw, peeled	1 lemon	17	trace	trace
Lemon juice				
Raw	1 lemon	12	0	0
Canned or bottled	1 cup	51	1	0.1
	1 tbsp.	3	trace	trace
Lime juice				
Raw	1 lime	10	trace	trace
Canned	1 cup	52	1	0.1
	1 tbsp.	3	trace	trace
Mangoes, raw, skinned, and seeded				
Whole	1 mango	135	1	0.1
Sliced	1 cup	107	trace	0.1
Nectarines				
Raw (2½" diameter)	1 nectarine	67	1	0.1
Oranges				
Whole	1 orange	62	trace	trace
Sections	1 cup	85	trace	trace
Orange juice	1 cup	112	trace	0.1

FAT AND CALORIE CHART

FOOD	AMOUNT	CALORIES	FAT (G)	SATURATED FAT (G)
Papayas, raw				
½" cubes	1 cup	55	trace	0.1
Whole	1 papaya	119	trace	0.1
Peaches				
Raw				
Whole	1 peach	42	trace	trace
Sliced	1 cup	73	trace	trace
Canned				
Heavy syrup	1 cup	194	trace	trace
Dried, sulfured	3 halves	93	trace	trace
Frozen	1 cup	235	trace	trace
Pears				
Raw	1 pear	98	1	trace
Canned, fruit and liquid				
Heavy syrup pack	1 cup	197	trace	trace
Pineapple				
Raw, diced	1 cup	76	1	trace
Canned, fruit and liquid				
Slices (3" diameter)	1 slice	38	trace	trace
Pineapple juice, unsweetened	1 cup	140	trace	trace
Plantain, peeled				
Raw	1 medium	218	1	0.3
Cooked, slices	1 cup	179	trace	0.1
Plums				
Raw (2-⅛" diameter)	1 plum	36	trace	trace
Canned, purple, fruit and liquid				
Heavy syrup pack	1 cup	230	trace	trace
	1 plum	41	trace	trace
Prunes, dried, pitted				
Uncooked	5 prunes	10	trace	trace
Stewed	1 cup	265	1	trace

FOOD	AMOUNT	CALORIES	FAT (G)	SATURATED FAT (G)
Prune juice, canned or bottled	1 cup	182	trace	trace
Raisins, seedless				
Not packed	1 cup	435	1	0.2
Packed	½ oz.	42	trace	trace
Raspberries				
Raw	1 cup	60	1	trace
Frozen	1 cup	258	trace	trace
Rhubarb, cooked with sugar	1 cup	278	trace	trace
Strawberries				
Large	1 strawberry	5	trace	trace
Medium	1 strawberry	4	trace	trace
Sliced	1 cup	50	1	trace
Frozen	1 cup	245	trace	trace
Tangerines, raw	1 tangerine	37	trace	trace
Canned (mandarin) oranges, light syrup, fruit and liquid				
	1 cup	154	trace	trace
Watermelon, diced	1 cup	49	1	0.1

GRAIN PRODUCTS

BAGELS, ENRICHED

FOOD	AMOUNT	CALORIES	FAT (G)	SATURATED FAT (G)
Plain	3½" bagel	195	1	0.2
	4" bagel	245	1	0.2
Cinnamon raisin	3½" bagel	195	1	0.2
	4" bagel	244	2	0.2
Egg	3½" bagel	197	1	0.3
	4" bagel	247	2	0.4
Banana bread	1 slice	196	6	1.3
Biscuits, plain or buttermilk, enriched				
	2½" biscuit	212	10	2.6
	4" biscuit	358	16	4.4

FAT AND CALORIE CHART

FOOD	AMOUNT	CALORIES	FAT (G)	SATURATED FAT (G)
BREADS				
Enriched				
Cracked wheat	1 slice	65	1	0.2
Egg bread (challah)	½" slice	115	2	0.6
French or Vienna (also sourdough)				
	½" slice	69	1	0.2
Italian	1 slice	54	1	0.2
Mixed grain bread	1 slice	65	1	0.2
Oatmeal	1 slice	73	1	0.2
Pita	4" pita	77	trace	trace
	6 ½" pita	165	1	0.1
Pumpernickel	1 slice	80	1	0.1
Raisin	1 slice	71	1	0.3
Rye	1 slice	83	1	0.2
Reduced-calorie	1 slice	47	1	0.1
Wheat	1 slice	65	1	0.2
Reduced-calorie	1 slice	46	1	0.1
White	1 slice	67	1	0.1
Soft crumbs	1 cup	120	2	0.2
Reduced-calorie	1 slice	48	1	0.1
Whole wheat	1 slice	69	1	0.3
BREAD CRUMBS				
Dry, grated				
Plain, enriched	1 cup	427	6	1.3
Seasoned, unenriched	1 cup	440	3	0.9
Bread stuffing, prepared from dry mix				
	½ cup	178	9	1.7

FOOD	AMOUNT	CALORIES	FAT (G)	SATURATED FAT (G)
BROWNIES				
Regular, large	1 brownie	227	9	2.4
Fat-free, 2" sq.	1 brownie	89	trace	0.2
Reduced-calorie, 2" sq.	1 brownie	84	2	1.1
Buckwheat flour, whole groat	1 cup	402	4	0.8
Buckwheat groats, roasted (kasha), cooked				
	1 cup	155	1	0.2
BULGUR				
Uncooked	1 cup	479	2	0.3
Cooked	1 cup	151	trace	0.1
CAKES				
Cakes, prepared from dry mix				
Angel food (1/12 of 10" cake)	1 piece	129	trace	trace
Yellow, light, with water, egg whites, no frosting (1/12 of 9" diameter)				
	1 piece	181	2	1.1
Cakes, prepared from recipe				
Chocolate, without frosting (1/12 of 9" diameter)				
	1 piece	340	14	5.2
Gingerbread (1/9 of 8" square)	1 piece	263	12	3.1
Pineapple upside down (1/9 of 8" square)				
	1 piece	367	14	3.4
Shortcake, biscuit type (about 3" diameter)				
	1 shortcake	225	9	2.5
Sponge (1/12 of 16-oz. cake)				
	1 piece	187	3	0.8
White without frosting (1/12 of 9" diameter)				
	1 piece	264	9	2
Cakes, commercially prepared				
Angel food (1/12 of 12-oz. cake)	1 piece	72	trace	trace

FAT AND CALORIE CHART

FOOD	AMOUNT	CALORIES	FAT (G)	SATURATED FAT (G)
Boston cream (1/6 of pie)	1 piece	232	8	2.2
Chocolate with chocolate frosting (1/8 of 18-oz. cake)				
	1 piece	235	10	3.1
Coffeecake, crumb (1/9 of 20-oz. cake)				
	1 piece	263	15	3.7
Fruitcake	1 piece	139	4	0.5
Pound				
Butter (1 1/12 of 12-oz. cake)	1 piece	109	6	3.2
Fat-free (3¼" x 2¾" x 5/8" slice)	1 slice	79	trace	0.1
Snack cakes				
Sponge	1 shortcake	87	1	0.2
Yellow				
With chocolate frosting	1 piece	243	11	3
With vanilla frosting	1 piece	239	9	1.5
Cheesecake (1/6 of 17-oz. cake)	1 piece	257	18	7.9

COOKIES

FOOD	AMOUNT	CALORIES	FAT (G)	SATURATED FAT (G)
Butter, commercially prepared	1 cookie	23	1	0.6
Chocolate chip, medium (2¼"-2½" diameter)				
Commercially prepared	1 cookie	48	2	0.7
From refrigerated dough	1 cookie	128	6	2
Prepared from recipe, with margarine				
	1 cookie	78	5	1.3
Fig bar	1 cookie	56	1	0.2
Molasses				
Medium	1 cookie	65	2	0.5
Large	1 cookie	138	4	1
Oatmeal				
Commercially prepared, with or without raisins				
Regular, large	1 cookie	113	5	1.1
Soft-type	1 cookie	61	2	0.5
Fat-free	1 cookie	36	trace	trace

FOOD	AMOUNT	CALORIES	FAT (G)	SATURATED FAT (G)
Prepared from recipe, with raisins (2⁵⁄₈" diameter)				
	1 cookie	65	2	0.5
Peanut butter				
Commercially prepared	1 cookie	72	4	0.7
Prepared from recipe, with margarine (3" diameter)				
	1 cookie	95	5	0.9
Sandwich-type, with cream filling				
Chocolate	1 cookie	47	2	0.4
Vanilla cookie, oval	1 cookie	72	3	0.4
Shortbread, commercially prepared				
Plain (1⁵⁄₈" square)	1 cookie	40	2	0.5
Pecan				
Regular (2")	1 cookie	76	5	1.1
Reduced fat	1 cookie	73	3	0.6
Sugar				
Commercially prepared	1 cookie	72	3	0.8
From refrigerated dough	1 cookie	73	3	0.9
Prepared from recipe, with margarine (3" diameter)				
	1 cookie	66	3	0.7
Vanilla wafer, lower-fat, medium size				
	1 cookie	18	1	0.2
CORN CHIPS				
Plain	1 oz.	153	9	1.3
CORNBREAD				
Prepared from mix	1 piece	188	6	1.6
COUSCOUS				
Uncooked	1 cup	650	1	0.2
Cooked	1 cup	176	trace	trace

FAT AND CALORIE CHART

FOOD	AMOUNT	CALORIES	FAT (G)	SATURATED FAT (G)
CRACKERS				
Cheese, 1" diameter	10 crackers	50	3	0.9
Graham, plain				
2½" square	2 squares	59	1	0.2
Crushed	1 cup	355	8	1.3
Melba toast, plain	4 pieces	78	1	0.1
Saltine				
Square	4 crackers	52	1	0.4
Oyster-type	1 cup	195	5	1.3
Standard snack type				
Bite size	1 cup	311	16	2.3
Round	4 crackers	60	3	0.5
Wheat, square	4 crackers	38	2	0.4
Whole wheat	4 crackers	71	3	0.5
DANISH PASTRY, ENRICHED				
Cheese-filled	1 Danish	266	16	4.8
Fruit-filled	1 Danish	263	13	3.5
DOUGHNUTS				
Cake-type	1 hole	59	3	0.5
	1 medium	198	11	1.7
Yeast leavened, glazed	1 hole	52	3	0.8
	1 medium	242	14	3.5
Éclair	1 éclair	262	16	4.1
ENGLISH MUFFIN	1 muffin	134	1	0.1
FRENCH TOAST				
Prepared from recipe	1 slice	149	7	1.8

FOOD	AMOUNT	CALORIES	FAT (G)	SATURATED FAT (G)
GRANOLA BAR				
Hard, plain	1 bar	134	6	0.7
Soft, uncoated chocolate chip	1 bar	119	5	2.9
Raisin	1 bar	127	5	2.7
MATZO				
Plain	1 matzo	112	trace	0.1
MUFFINS (2½" X 2¼")				
Blueberry				
Commercially prepared	1 muffin	158	4	0.8
Prepared from recipe	1 muffin	162	6	1.2
Bran with raisins				
Toasted	1 muffin	106	3	0.5
Corn				
Commercially prepared	1 muffin	174	5	0.8
Prepared from mix	1 muffin	161	5	1.4
Oat bran, commercially prepared				
	1 muffin	154	4	0.6
NOODLES				
Egg noodles, enriched, cooked				
Regular	1 cup	213	2	0.5
Spinach	1 cup	211	3	0.6
Macaroni (elbows), enriched, cooked				
	1 cup	197	1	0.1
OAT BRAN				
Uncooked	1 cup	231	7	1.2
Cooked	1 cup	88	2	0.4

FAT AND CALORIE CHART

FOOD	AMOUNT	CALORIES	FAT (G)	SATURATED FAT (G)
PANCAKES, PLAIN (4" DIAMETER)				
Prepared from complete mix				
	1 pancake	74	1	0.2
Prepared from incomplete mix, with 2% milk, egg, and oil				
	1 pancake	83	3	0.8
PIES				
Prepared from recipe (⅛ of 9" diameter)				
Apple	1 piece	411	19	4.7
Blueberry	1 piece	360	17	4.3
Cherry	1 piece	486	22	5.4
Lemon meringue	1 piece	362	16	4
Pecan	1 piece	503	27	4.9
Pumpkin	1 piece	316	14	4.9
Fried, cherry	1 pie	404	21	3.1
POPCORN				
Air-popped, plain	1 cup	31	trace	trace
Oil-popped, salted	1 cup	55	3	0.5
Caramel-coated				
with peanuts	1 cup	168	3	0.4
without peanuts	1 cup	152	5	1.3
Cheese-flavored	1 cup	58	4	0.7
Popcorn cake	1 cake	38	trace	trace
PRETZELS, MADE WITH ENRICHED FLOUR				
Stick, 2¼" long	10 pretzels	11	trace	trace
Twisted, regular	10 pretzels	229	2	0.5
Twisted, Dutch	1 pretzel	61	1	0.1

FOOD	AMOUNT	CALORIES	FAT (G)	SATURATED FAT (G)
RICE				
Brown, long grain, cooked	1 cup	216	2	0.4
Regular				
Raw	1 cup	675	1	0.3
Cooked	1 cup	205	trace	0.1
Instant, prepared	1 cup	162	trace	0.1
ROLLS				
Dinner	1 roll	84	2	0.5
Hamburger/hotdog	1 roll	123	2	0.5
Hard, Kaiser	1 roll	167	2	0.3
SPAGHETTI, COOKED				
Enriched	1 cup	197	1	0.1
Whole wheat	1 cup	174	1	0.1
SWEET ROLLS, CINNAMON				
Commercial, with raisins	1 roll	223	10	1.8
Refrigerated dough, baked, with frosting				
	1 roll	109	4	1
TACO SHELL, BAKED	1 medium	62	3	0.4
TAPIOCA, PEARL, DRY	1 cup	544	trace	trace
TORTILLA CHIPS				
Plain				
Regular	1 oz.	142	7	14
Low-fat, baked	10 chips	54	1	0.1

FAT AND CALORIE CHART

FOOD	AMOUNT	CALORIES	FAT (G)	SATURATED FAT (G)
WAFFLES, PLAIN				
Prepared from recipe, 7" diameter				
	1 waffle	218	11	2.1
Frozen, toasted, 4" diameter	1 waffle	87	3	0.5
WHEAT FLOURS				
All-purpose, enriched				
Sifted, spooned	1 cup	419	1	0.2
Unsifted, spooned	1 cup	455	1	0.2
Bread, enriched	1 cup	495	2	0.3
Cake or pastry flour, enriched, unsifted, spooned				
	1 cup	496	1	0.2
Self-rising, enriched, unsifted, spooned				
	1 cup	443	1	0.2
Whole wheat, from hard wheat, stirred, spooned				
	1 cup	407	2	0.4
Wheat germ, toasted, plain	1 tbsp.	27	2	0.1
LEGUMES, NUTS, AND SEEDS				
ALMONDS, SHELLED				
Sliced	1 cup	549	48	3.7
Whole	1 oz. (24 nuts)	164	14	1.1
BEANS, DRY				
Cooked				
Black	1 cup	227	1	0.2
Great Northern	1 cup	209	1	0.2
Kidney, red	1 cup	225	1	0.1
Lima, large	1 cup	216	1	0.2
Pea (navy)	1 cup	258	1	0.3
Pinto	1 cup	234	1	0.2

FOOD	AMOUNT	CALORIES	FAT (G)	SATURATED FAT (G)
Canned, solids and liquid				
Baked beans				
Plain or vegetarian	1 cup	236	1	0.3
With pork in tomato sauce	1 cup	248	3	1
With pork in sweet sauce	1 cup	281	4	1.4
Kidney, red	1 cup	218	1	0.1
Lima, large	1 cup	190	trace	0.1
White	1 cup	307	1	0.2
Black-eyed peas				
Cooked	1 cup	20	1	0.2
Canned, solids and liquid	1 cup	185	1	0.3
Brazil nuts, shelled 1 oz. (6-8 nuts)		186	19	4.6
Cashews, salted				
Dry-roasted	1 oz.	163	13	2.6
Oil-roasted	1 cup	749	63	12.4
Chestnuts, European, roasted, shelled				
	1 cup	350	3	0.6
Chickpeas				
Cooked	1 cup	269	4	0.4
Canned, solids and liquid	1 cup	286	3	0.3
Coconut				
Raw				
Piece, about 2" x 2" x ½"	1 piece	159	15	13.4
Shredded, not packed	1 cup	283	27	23.8
Dried, sweetened, shredded	1 cup	466	33	29.3
Hazelnuts (filberts), chopped	1 cup	722	70	5.1
Hummus, prepared	1 tbsp.	23	1	0.2
Lentils, dry, cooked	1 cup	230	1	0.1
Macadamia nuts, dry-roasted, salted				
	1 cup	959	102	16

FAT AND CALORIE CHART

FOOD	AMOUNT	CALORIES	FAT (G)	SATURATED FAT (G)
Mixed nuts, with peanuts, salted				
Dry-roasted	1 oz.	168	15	2
Oil-roasted	1 oz.	175	16	2.5
Peanuts				
Dry-roasted				
Salted	1 oz. (about 28)	166	14	2
Unsalted	1 oz. (about 28)	166	14	2
Oil-roasted, salted	1 oz.	165	14	1.9
Peanut butter				
Regular				
Smooth-style	1 tbsp.	95	8	1.7
Chunk-style	1 tbsp.	94	8	1.5
Reduced-fat	1 tbsp.	94	6	1.3
Peas, split, dry, cooked	1 cup	231	1	0.1
Pecans, halves	1 cup	746	78	6.7
Pine nuts, shelled	1 oz.	160	14	2.2
Pistachio nuts, dry-roasted, with salt, shelled				
	1 oz. (47 nuts)	161	13	1.6
Pumpkin and squash kernels, roasted, with salt				
	1 oz.	148	12	2.3
Refried beans, canned	1 cup	237	3	1.2
Sesame seeds	1 tbsp.	47	4	0.6
Soybeans, dry, cooked	1 cup	298	15	2.2
Soy products				
Soy milk	1 cup	81	5	0.5
Tofu				
Firm	¼ block	62	4	0.5
Soft, piece 2½" x ½" x 1"	1 piece	73	4	0.6
Sunflower seed kernels, dry-roasted, with salt				
	¼ cup	186	16	1.7
	1 oz.	165	14	1.5

FOOD	AMOUNT	CALORIES	FAT (G)	SATURATED FAT (G)
Tahini	1 tbsp.	89	8	1.1
Walnuts, English	1 cup	785	78	7.4

MEAT AND MEAT PRODUCTS
BEEF, COOKED
Cuts braised, simmered, or pot-roasted

Relatively fat, such as chuck blade, piece, 2½" x 2½" x ¾"

Lean and fat	3 oz.	293	22	8.7
Lean only	3 oz.	213	11	4.3

Relatively lean, such as bottom round, piece, 4⅛" x 2¼" x ½"

Lean and fat	3 oz.	234	14	5.4
Lean only	3 oz.	178	7	2.4

Ground beef, broiled

83% lean	3 oz.	218	14	5.5
79% lean	3 oz.	231	16	6.2
73% lean	3 oz.	246	18	6.9

Roast, oven cooked, no liquid added

Relatively fat, such as rib, 2 pieces, 4⅛" x 2¼" x ¼"

Lean and fat	3 oz.	304	25	9.9
Lean only	3 oz.	195	11	4.2

Relatively lean, such as eye of round, 2 pieces, 2½" x 2½" x 3/8"

Lean and fat	3 oz.	195	11	4.2
Lean only	3 oz.	143	4	1.5

Steak, sirloin, broiled, piece, 2½" x 2½" x ¾"

Lean and fat	3 oz.	219	13	5.2
Lean only	3 oz.	166	6	2.4

LAMB, COOKED
Chops

Loin, broiled

Lean and fat	3 oz.	269	20	8.4
Lean only	3 oz.	184	8	3

FAT AND CALORIE CHART

FOOD	AMOUNT	CALORIES	FAT (G)	SATURATED FAT (G)
Leg, roasted, 2 pieces, 4⅛" x 2¼" x ¼"				
Lean and fat	3 oz.	219	14	5.9
Lean only	3 oz.	162	7	2.3
Rib, roasted, 3 pieces, 2½" x 2½" x ¼"				
Lean and fat	3 oz.	305	25	10.9
Lean only	3 oz.	197	11	4
PORK, CURED, COOKED				
Bacon				
Regular	3 slices	109	9	3.3
Canadian style (6 slices per 6-oz. pack.)				
	2 slices	86	4	1.3
Ham, light cure, roasted, 2 pieces, 4⅛" x 2¼" x ¼"				
Lean and fat	3 oz.	207	14	5.1
Lean only	3 oz.	133	5	1.6
Pork, fresh, cooked				
Broiled				
Lean and fat	3 oz.	204	11	4.1
Lean only	3 oz.	172	7	2.5
Pan-fried				
Lean and fat	3 oz.	235	14	5.1
Lean only	3 oz.	197	9	3.1
Ham (leg), roasted, piece, 2½" x 2½" x ¾"				
Lean and fat	3 oz.	232	15	5.5
Lean only	3 oz.	179	8	2.8
Rib roast, piece, 2½" x 2½" x ¾"				
Lean and fat	3 oz.	217	13	5
Lean only	3 oz.	190	9	3.7
Ribs, lean and fat, cooked				
Backribs, roasted	3 oz.	315	25	9.3
Country-style, braised	3 oz.	252	18	6.8
Spareribs, braised	3 oz.	337	26	9.5

FOOD	AMOUNT	CALORIES	FAT (G)	SATURATED FAT (G)
Shoulder cut, braised, 3 pieces, 2½" x 2½" x ¼"				
Lean and fat	3 oz.	280	20	7.2
Lean only	3 oz.	211	10	3.5

SAUSAGES

FOOD	AMOUNT	CALORIES	FAT (G)	SATURATED FAT (G)
Bologna, beef and pork (8 slices per 8-oz. pack)				
	2 slices	180	16	6.1
Brown and serve, cooked, link, 4" x 7⁄8" raw				
	2 links	103	9	3.4
Frankfurter (10 per 1-lb. pack), heated				
Beef and pork	1 frank	144	13	4.8
Beef	1 frank	142	13	5.4
Pork sausage, fresh, cooked				
Link	2 links	96	8	2.8
Patty	1 patty	10	8	2.9
Salami, beef and pork				
Cooked type (8 slices per 8-oz. pack)				
	2 slices	143	11	4.6
Dry type, sliced, 3⅛" x 1⁄16"	2 slices	84	7	2.4
Vienna sausage (7 per 4-oz. can)				
	1 sausage	45	4	1.5

FAST FOODS

FOOD	AMOUNT	CALORIES	FAT (G)	SATURATED FAT (G)
Breakfast items				
Biscuit with egg, sausage	1 biscuit	581	39	15
Croissant with egg, cheese, bacon				
	1 croissant	413	28	15.4
Danish pastry				
Cheese-filled	1 pastry	353	25	5.1
Fruit-filled	1 pastry	335	16	3.3

FAT AND CALORIE CHART

FOOD	AMOUNT	CALORIES	FAT (G)	SATURATED FAT (G)
English muffin with egg, cheese, Canadian bacon				
	1 muffin	289	13	4.7
French toast with butter	2 slices	356	19	7.7
French toast sticks	5 sticks	513	29	4.7
Hashed brown potatoes	½ cup	151	9	4.3
Pancakes with butter, syrup	2 pancakes	520	14	5.9
Burrito				
Beans and cheese	1 burrito	189	6	3.4
Beans and meat	1 burrito	255	9	4.2
Cheeseburger				
Regular size, with condiments				
Double patty with mayo-type dressing, vegetables				
	1 sandwich	417	21	8.7
Single patty	1 sandwich	295	14	6.3
Single patty with bacon	1 sandwich	608	37	16.2
Chicken fillet (breaded and fried) sandwich, plain				
	1 sandwich	515	29	8.5
CHICKEN, FRIED: See Poultry and Poultry Products				
Chicken pieces, boneless, breaded and fried, plain				
	6 pieces	319	21	4.7
Chili con carne	1 cup	256	8	3.4
Chimichanga with beef	1 chimichanga	425	20	8.5
Coleslaw	¾ cup	147	11	1.6
Enchilada with cheese	1 enchilada	319	19	10.6
Fish sandwich, with tartar sauce and cheese				
	1 sandwich	523	29	8.1
French fries	1 small	291	16	3.3
	1 medium	458	25	5.2
	1 large	578	31	6.5

FOOD	AMOUNT	CALORIES	FAT (G)	SATURATED FAT (G)
Hamburger				
Regular size, with condiments				
Double patty	1 sandwich	576	32	12
Single patty	1 sandwich	272	10	3.6
Hot dog				
Corndog	1 corndog	460	19	5.2
Plain	1 sandwich	242	15	5.1
With chili	1 sandwich	296	13	4.9
Onion rings, breaded and fried	8-9 rings	276	16	7
Pizza (slice = 1/8 of 12" pizza)				
Cheese	1 slice	140	3	1.5
Meat and vegetables	1 slice	184	5	1.5
Pepperoni	1 slice	181	7	2.2
Shake				
Chocolate	16 fl. oz.	423	12	7.7
Vanilla	16 fl. oz.	370	10	6.2
Shrimp, breaded and fried	6-8 shrimp	454	25	5.4
Submarine sandwich (6"), with oil and vinegar				
Cold cuts (with lettuce, cheese, salami, ham, tomato, onion)				
	1 sandwich	456	19	6.8
Roast beef (with tomato, lettuce, mayo)				
	1 sandwich	410	13	7.1
Tuna salad (with mayo, lettuce)				
	1 sandwich	584	28	5.3
Taco, beef	1 small	369	21	11.4

POULTRY AND POULTRY PRODUCTS
CHICKEN

Fried in vegetable shortening, meat with skin

Batter-dipped				
Breast	½ breast	364	18	4.9

FAT AND CALORIE CHART

FOOD	AMOUNT	CALORIES	FAT (G)	SATURATED FAT (G)
Drumstick	1 drumstick	193	11	3
Thigh	1 thigh	238	14	3.8
Wing	1 wing	159	11	2.9
Flour-coated				
Breast	½ breast	218	9	2.4
Drumstick	1 drumstick	120	7	1.8
Fried, meat only				
Dark meat	3 oz.	203	10	2.7
Light meat	3 oz.	163	5	1.3
Roasted, meat only				
Breast	½ breast	142	3	0.9
Drumstick	1 drumstick	76	2	0.7
Thigh	1 thigh	109	6	1.6
Stewed, meat only, light and dark meat, chopped or diced				
	1 cup	332	17	4.3
DUCK				
Roasted, flesh only	½ duck	444	25	9.2
TURKEY				
Roasted, meat only				
Dark meat	3 oz.	159	6	2.1
Light meat	3 oz.	133	3	0.9
SOUPS, SAUCES, AND GRAVIES				
SOUPS				
Home-prepared stock				
Beef	1 cup	31	trace	0.1
Chicken	1 cup	86	3	0.8
Fish	1 cup	40	2	0.5

FOOD	AMOUNT	CALORIES	FAT (G)	SATURATED FAT (G)
SAUCES				
Ready-to-serve				
Barbecue	1 tbsp.	12	trace	trace
Cheese	¼ cup	110	8	3.8
Hoisin	1 tbsp.	35	1	0.1
Nacho cheese	¼ cup	119	10	4.2
Pepper or hot	1 tsp.	90	trace	trace
Salsa	1 tbsp.	4	trace	trace
Soy	1 tbsp.	9	trace	trace
Spaghetti/marinara/pasta	1 cup	143	5	0.7
Teriyaki	1 tbsp.	15	0	0
Tomato chili	¼ cup	71	trace	trace
Worcestershire	1 tbsp.	11	0	0
Gravies, canned				
Beef	¼ cup	31	1	0.7
Chicken	¼ cup	47	3	0.8
Country sausage	¼ cup	96	8	2
Mushroom	¼ cup	30	2	0.2
Turkey	¼ cup	31	1	0.4
SUGARS AND SWEETS				
CANDY				
Caramel				
Plain	1 piece	39	1	0.7
Chocolate-flavored	1 piece	25	trace	trace
Carob	1 oz.	153	9	8.2
Chocolate chips				
Milk	1 cup	862	52	31
Semisweet	1 cup	805	50	29.8
White	1 cup	916	55	33
Chocolate-coated peanuts	10 pieces	208	13	5.8

FAT AND CALORIE CHART

FOOD	AMOUNT	CALORIES	FAT (G)	SATURATED FAT (G)
Chocolate-coated raisins	10 pieces	39	1	0.9
Fruit leather, rolls	1 large	74	1	0.1
	1 small	49	trace	0.1
Fudge, prepared from recipe				
Chocolate	1 piece	65	1	0.9
Vanilla	1 piece	59	1	0.5
Gumdrops/gummy candies				
Gumdrops (¾")	1 cup	703	0	0
Gummy bears	10 bears	85	0	0
Hard candy	1 piece	24	trace	0
Jelly beans	10 large	104	trace	trace
Marshmallows				
Miniature	1 cup	159	trace	trace
Regular	1 regular	23	trace	trace
Frosting, ready-to-eat				
Chocolate	1/12 package	151	7	2.1
Vanilla	1/12 package	159	6	1.9
Frozen desserts (nondairy)				
Fruit and juice bar	1 bar (2.5 fl. oz.)	63	trace	0
Ice pop	1 bar (2 fl. oz.)	42	0	0
Italian ices	½ cup	86	trace	0
Gelatin dessert, prepared with gelatin dessert powder and water				
Regular	½ cup	80	0	0
Reduced calorie (with aspartame)				
	½ cup	8	0	0
Honey, strained or extracted	1 tbsp.	64	0	0
Jams and preserves	1 tbsp.	56	trace	trace
Jellies	1 tbsp.	54	trace	trace
Puddings				
Chocolate	½ cup	150	3	1.6
Vanilla	½ cup	148	2	1.4

FOOD	AMOUNT	CALORIES	FAT (G)	SATURATED FAT (G)
Sugar				
Brown				
Packed	1 cup	827	0	0
Unpacked	1 cup	545	0	0
White				
Granulated	1 packet	23	0	0
	1 tsp.	16	0	0
Powdered, unsifted	1 tbsp.	31	trace	trace
Syrup				
Chocolate-flavored syrup or topping				
Thin type	1 tbsp.	53	trace	0.1
Fudge type	1 tbsp.	67	2	0.8
Corn, light	1 tbsp.	56	0	0
Maple	1 tbsp.	52	trace	trace
Molasses, blackstrap	1 tbsp.	47	0	0
Table blend, pancake				
Regular	1 tbsp.	57	0	0
VEGETABLES AND VEGETABLE PRODUCTS				
Alfalfa sprouts, raw	1 cup	10	trace	trace
Artichokes, globe or French, cooked, drained				
	1 cup	84	trace	0.1
	1 medium	60	trace	trace
Asparagus, green				
Cooked, drained				
From raw	1 cup	43	1	0.1
	4 spears	14	trace	trace
From frozen	1 cup	50	1	0.2
	4 spears	17	trace	0.1
Canned, spears about 5" long, drained				
	1 cup	46	2	0.4
	4 spears	14	trace	0.1

FAT AND CALORIE CHART

FOOD	AMOUNT	CALORIES	FAT (G)	SATURATED FAT (G)
Bamboo shoots, canned, drained	1 cup	25	1	0.1
BEANS				
Lima, immature seeds, frozen, cooked, drained				
Fordhooks	1 cup	170	1	0.1
Baby limas	1 cup	189	1	0.1
Snap, cut				
Cooked, drained				
From raw				
Green	1 cup	44	trace	0.1
Yellow	1 cup	44	trace	0.1
From frozen				
Green	1 cup	38	trace	0.1
Yellow	1 cup	38	trace	0.1
Canned, drained				
Green	1 cup	27	trace	trace
Yellow	1 cup	27	trace	trace
BEANS, DRY: See Legumes				
Bean sprouts (mung)				
Raw	1 cup	31	trace	trace
Cooked, drained	1 cup	26	trace	trace
Beets				
Cooked, drained				
Slices	1 cup	75	trace	trace
Whole beet, 2"	1 beet	22	trace	trace
Canned, drained				
Slices	1 cup	53	trace	trace
Whole beet	1 beet	7	trace	trace
Beet greens, leaves and stems, cooked, drained, 1" pieces				
	1 cup	89	trace	trace

FOOD	AMOUNT	CALORIES	FAT (G)	SATURATED FAT (G)
Black-eyed peas, immature seeds, cooked, drained				
From raw	1 cup	160	1	0.2
From frozen	1 cup	224	1	0.3
Broccoli				
Raw				
Chopped or diced	1 cup	25	trace	trace
Spear, 5" long	1 spear	9	trace	trace
Cooked, drained				
From raw				
Chopped	1 cup	44	1	0.1
Spear, 5" long	1 spear	10	trace	trace
From frozen, chopped	1 cup	52	trace	trace
Brussels sprouts, cooked, drained				
From raw	1 cup	61	1	0.2
From frozen	1 cup	65	1	0.1
Cabbage, common varieties, shredded				
Raw	1 cup	18	trace	trace
Cooked, drained	1 cup	33	1	0.1
Cabbage, Chinese, shredded, cooked, drained				
Pak choi / bok choy	1 cup	20	trace	trace
Pe-tsai	1 cup	17	trace	trace
Cabbage, red, raw, shredded	1 cup	19	trace	trace
Cabbage, Savoy, raw, shredded	1 cup	19	trace	trace
Carrot juice, canned	1 cup	94	trace	0.1
Carrots				
Raw				
Whole, 7½" long	1 carrot	31	trace	trace
Grated	1 cup	47	trace	trace
Baby	1 medium	4	trace	trace
Cooked, sliced, drained				
From raw	1 cup	70	trace	0.1
From frozen	1 cup	53	trace	trace

FAT AND CALORIE CHART

FOOD	AMOUNT	CALORIES	FAT (G)	SATURATED FAT (G)
Canned, sliced, drained	1 cup	37	trace	0.1
Cauliflower				
Raw	1 floweret	3	trace	trace
	1 cup	25	trace	trace
Celery				
Raw				
Stalk, 8" long	1 stalk	6	trace	trace
Pieces, diced	1 cup	19	trace	trace
Chives, raw	1 tbsp.	1	trace	trace
Cilantro, raw	1 tsp.	trace	trace	trace
Coleslaw, home-prepared	1 cup	83	3	0.5
Collards, cooked, drained, chopped				
From raw	1 cup	49	1	0.1
From frozen	1 cup	61	1	0.1
Corn, sweet, yellow				
Cooked, drained				
From raw cob	1 ear	83	1	0.2
From frozen				
Kernels on cob	1 ear	59	trace	0.1
Kernels	1 cup	131	1	0.1
Canned				
Cream style	1 cup	184	1	0.2
Whole kernel, vacuum pack	1 cup	166	1	0.2
Corn, sweet, white, cooked, drained	1 ear	83	1	0.2
Cucumber				
Peeled				
Sliced	1 cup	14	trace	trace
Whole, 8¼"	1 large	34	trace	0.1
Unpeeled				
Sliced	1 cup	14	trace	trace
Whole, 8¼"	1 large	39	trace	0.1

FOOD	AMOUNT	CALORIES	FAT (G)	SATURATED FAT (G)
Dandelion greens, cooked, drained				
	1 cup	35	1	0.2
Dill, raw	5 sprigs	trace	trace	trace
Eggplant, cooked, drained	1 cup	28	trace	trace
Endive, curly (including escarole), raw, small pieces				
	1 cup	9	trace	trace
Garlic, raw	1 clove	4	trace	trace
Hearts of palm, canned	1 piece	9	trace	trace
Jerusalem artichoke, raw, sliced	1 cup	114	trace	0
Kale, cooked, drained, chopped				
From raw	1 cup	36	1	0.1
From frozen	1 cup	39	1	0.1
Kohlrabi, cooked, drained, slices	1 cup	48	trace	trace
Leeks, bulb and lower leaf portion, chopped or diced, cooked, drained				
	1 cup	32	trace	trace
Lettuce, raw				
Butterhead, Boston types				
Leaf	1 medium leaf	1	trace	trace
Head, 5" diameter	1 head	21	trace	trace
Crisphead, as iceberg				
Leaf	1 medium	1	trace	trace
Head, 6" diameter	1 head	65	1	0.1
Pieces, shredded or chopped	1 cup	7	trace	trace
Loose leaf head				
Leaf	1 leaf	2	trace	trace
Pieces, shredded	1 cup	10	trace	trace
Romaine or Cos				
Innerleaf	1 leaf	1	trace	trace
Pieces, shredded	1 cup	8	trace	trace
Mushrooms				
Raw, cut up	1 cup	18	trace	trace

FAT AND CALORIE CHART

FOOD	AMOUNT	CALORIES	FAT (G)	SATURATED FAT (G)
Cooked, drained	1 cup	42	1	0.1
Canned, drained	1 cup	37	trace	0.1
Mushrooms, shiitake				
Cooked pieces	1 cup	80	trace	0.1
Dried	1 mushroom	11	trace	trace
Mustard greens, cooked, drained	1 cup	21	trace	trace
Okra, sliced, cooked, drained				
From raw	1 cup	51	trace	0.1
From frozen	1 cup	52	1	0.1
Onions				
Raw				
Chopped	1 cup	61	trace	trace
Whole, medium, 2½" diameter				
	1 whole	42	trace	trace
Slice, 1/8" thick	1 slice	5	trace	trace
Cooked (whole or sliced), drained				
	1 cup	92	trace	0.1
	1 medium	41	trace	trace
Dehydrated flakes	1 tbsp.	17	trace	trace
Onions, spring, raw, top and bulb				
Chopped	1 cup	32	trace	trace
Whole, medium, 4⅛" long	1 whole	5	trace	trace
Parsley, raw	10 sprigs	4	trace	trace
Parsnips, sliced, cooked, drained	1 cup	126	trace	0.1
Peas, edible pod, cooked, drained				
From raw	1 cup	67	trace	0.1
From frozen	1 cup	83	1	0.1
Peas, green				
Canned, drained	1 cup	117	1	0.1
Frozen	1 cup	125	trace	0.1

FOOD	AMOUNT	CALORIES	FAT (G)	SATURATED FAT (G)
Peppers				
Hot chili, raw				
Green	1 pepper	18	trace	trace
Red	1 pepper	18	trace	trace
Jalapeno, canned, sliced, solids and liquids				
	¼ cup	7	trace	trace
Sweet (2¾" long, 2½" diameter)				
Raw				
Green				
Chopped	1 cup	40	trace	trace
Ring (¼")	1 ring	3	trace	trace
Whole	1 pepper	32	trace	trace
Red				
Chopped	1 cup	40	trace	trace
Whole	1 pepper	32	trace	trace
Cooked, drained, chopped				
Green	1 cup	38	trace	trace
Red	1 cup	38	trace	trace
Pimento, canned	1 tbsp.	3	trace	trace
Potatoes				
Baked (2⅓" x 4¾")				
With skin	1 potato	220	trace	0.1
Flesh only	1 potato	145	trace	trace
Skin only	1 skin	115	trace	trace
Boiled (2½" diameter)				
Peeled after boiling	1 potato	118	trace	trace
Peeled before boiling	1 potato	116	trace	trace
	1 cup	134	trace	trace

FAT AND CALORIE CHART

FOOD	AMOUNT	CALORIES	FAT (G)	SATURATED FAT (G)
Potato products, prepared				
Au gratin				
From dry mix, with whole milk, butter				
	1 cup	228	10	6.3
From home recipe, with butter				
	1 cup	323	19	11.6
French-fried, frozen, oven-heated				
	10 strips	10	4	0.6
Hashed brown				
From frozen (about 3" x 1½" x ½")				
	1 patty	63	3	1.3
From home recipe	1 cup	326	22	8.5
Mashed				
From dehydrated flakes; whole milk, butter and salt added				
	1 cup	237	12	7.2
From home recipe				
With whole milk	1 cup	162	1	0.7
With whole milk and margarine				
	1 cup	223	9	2.2
Potato pancakes, home-prepared				
	1 pancake	207	12	2.3
Potato puffs, from frozen	10 puffs	175	8	4
Potato salad, home-prepared	1 cup	358	21	3.6
Scalloped				
From dry mix, with whole milk, butter				
	1 cup	228	11	6.5
From home recipe, with butter				
	1 cup	211	9	5.5
Pumpkin				
Cooked, mashed	1 cup	49	trace	0.1
Canned	1 cup	83	1	0.4

FOOD	AMOUNT	CALORIES	FAT (G)	SATURATED FAT (G)
Radishes, raw	1 radish	1	trace	trace
Rutabagas, cooked	1 cup	66	trace	trace
Sauerkraut, canned, solids and liquid				
	1 cup	45	race	0.1
Seaweed				
Kelp, raw	2 tbsp.	4	trace	trace
Spirulina, dried	1 tbsp.	3	trace	trace
Shallots, chopped	1 tbsp.	7	trace	trace
Soybeans, green, cooked, drained	1 cup	254	12	1.3
Spinach				
Raw				
Chopped	1 cup	7	trace	trace
Leaf	1 leaf	2	trace	trace
Cooked, drained				
From raw	1 cup	41	trace	0.1
From frozen (chopped or leaf)	1 cup	53	trace	0.1
Canned, drained	1 cup	49	1	0.2
Squash				
Summer (all varieties), sliced				
Raw	1 cup	23	trace	trace
Cooked, drained	1 cup	36	1	0.1
Winter (all varieties), baked, cubes				
	1 cup	80	1	0.3
Winter, butternut, frozen, cooked, mashed				
	1 cup	94	trace	trace
Sweet potatoes				
Cooked (2" diameter, 5" long raw)				
Baked, with skin	1 potato	150	trace	trace
Boiled, without skin	1 potato	164	race	0.1
Candied (2½" x 2" piece)	1 piece	144	3	1.4

FAT AND CALORIE CHART

FOOD	AMOUNT	CALORIES	FAT (G)	SATURATED FAT (G)
Canned				
Syrup pack, drained	1 cup	212	1	0.1
Vacuum pack, mashed	1 cup	232	1	0.1
Tomatillos, raw	1 medium	11	trace	trace
Tomatoes				
Raw, year-round average				
Chopped or sliced	1 cup	38	1	0.1
	¼" slice	4	trace	trace
Whole				
Cherry	1 cherry	4	trace	trace
Medium, 2³⁄₅" diameter	1 tomato	26	trace	0.1
Canned, solids and liquid	1 cup	46	trace	trace
Sun-dried				
Plain	1 piece	5	trace	trace
Packed in oil, drained	1 piece	6	trace	0.1
Tomato juice, canned, salt added	1 cup	41	trace	trace
Tomato products, canned				
Paste	1 cup	215	1	0.2
Purée	1 cup	10	trace	0.1
Sauce	1 cup	74	trace	0.1
Stewed	1 cup	71	trace	trace
Turnips, cooked	1 cup	33	trace	trace
Turnip greens, cooked, drained				
From raw	1 cup	29	trace	0.1
From frozen	1 cup	49	1	0.2
Vegetable juice cocktail, canned	1 cup	46	trace	trace
Vegetables, mixed				
Canned, drained	1 cup	77	trace	0.1
Frozen, cooked,	1 cup	107	trace	0.1
Water chestnuts, canned, slices, solids and liquids				
	1 cup	70	trace	trace

FOOD	AMOUNT	CALORIES	FAT (G)	SATURATED FAT (G)
MISCELLANEOUS ITEMS				
Mustard, yellow	1 tsp.	3	trace	trace
Olives, canned				
Pickled, green	5 medium	20	2	0.3
Ripe, black	5 large	25	2	0.3
Pickles, cucumber				
Dill, whole, medium	1 pickle	12	trace	trace
Bread-and-butter slices, 1 ½" diameter, ¼" thick				
	3 slices	18	trace	trace
Pickle relish, sweet	1 tbsp.	20	trace	trace
Pork skins/rinds, plain	1 oz.	155	9	3.2
Potato chips				
Regular				
Plain				
Salted	1 oz.	152	10	3.1
Unsalted	1 oz.	152	10	3.1
Barbecue flavor	1 oz.	139	9	2.3
Sour cream and onion-flavored				
	1 oz.	151	10	2.5
Reduced-fat	1 oz.	134	6	1.2
Fat-free, with Olestra	1 oz.	75	trace	trace
Made from dried potatoes				
Plain	1 oz.	158	11	2.7
Sour cream and onion-flavored				
	1 oz.	155	10	2.7
Reduced-fat	1 oz.	142	7	1.5
Trail mix				
Regular, with raisins, chocolate chips, salted nuts, and seeds				
	1 cup	707	47	8.9
Tropical	1 cup	570	24	11.9

ESSENTIAL VITAMINS AND MINERALS
FIVE GREAT SOURCES FOR YOUR DAILY ESSENTIALS[4]

DIETARY FIBER

The recommended daily allowance for adult women is 25 grams.

FOOD	AMOUNT	DIETARY FIBER (G)
Navy beans, cooked	½ cup	9.5
Split peas, cooked	½ cup	8.1
Lentils, cooked	½ cup	7.8
Lima beans, cooked	½ cup	6.6
Artichoke, cooked	1 globe	6.5

CALCIUM

The recommended daily allowance for adults is 1,000 milligrams.

FOOD	AMOUNT	CALCIUM (MG)
Plain yogurt, non-fat	8 oz.	452
Romano cheese	1.5 oz.	452
Swiss cheese	1.5 oz.	335
Provolone cheese	1.5 oz.	321
Cheddar cheese	1.5 oz.	307

4. Information taken from "Dietary Guidelines for Americans 2005"
    U.S. Department of Health and Human Services
    U.S. Department of Agriculture
    www.healthierus.gov/dietaryguidelines

IRON

The recommended daily allowance for teen and adult females is 18 milligrams.

FOOD	AMOUNT	IRON (MG)
Clams, canned, drained	3 oz.	23.8
Oysters, eastern wild, cooked	3 oz.	10.2
Soybeans, mature, cooked	½ cup	4.4
Pumpkin and squash seed kernels, roasted	1 oz.	4.2
White beans, canned	½ cup	3.9

POTASSIUM

The recommended daily allowance for adults is 4,700 milligrams.

FOOD	AMOUNT	POTASSIUM (MG)
Sweet potato, baked	1 potato (146 g)	694
Beet greens, cooked	½ cup	655
Potato, baked, flesh	1 potato (156 g)	610
White beans, canned	½ cup	595
Yogurt, plain, non-fat	8 oz.	579

VITAMIN A

The recommended daily allowance of Vitamin A for adult men is 900 micrograms.

FOOD	AMOUNT	VITAMIN A (MICROGRAMS)
Carrot juice	¾ cup	1,692
Sweet potato w/peel, baked	1 medium	1,096
Pumpkin, canned	½ cup	953
Carrots, cooked from fresh	½ cup	671
Spinach, cooked from frozen	½ cup	573

VITAMIN C

The recommended daily allowance of Vitamin C for adult men is 90 milligrams.

FOOD	AMOUNT	VITAMIN C (MG)
Guava, raw	½ cup	188
Red sweet pepper, raw	½ cup	142
Kiwi fruit	1 medium	70
Orange juice	¾ cup	61–93
Grapefruit juice	¾ cup	50–70

VITAMIN E

The recommended daily allowance of Vitamin E for adults is 15 milligrams.

FOOD	AMOUNT	VITAMIN E (MG)
Sunflower seeds, dry roasted	1 oz.	7.4
Almonds	1 oz.	7.3
Sunflower oil	1 tbsp.	5.6
Hazelnuts (filberts)	1 oz.	4.3
Mixed nuts, dry-roasted	1 oz.	3.1

NOTES